Gathering of Kindness

ANTHOLOGY

Edited by Mish Phillips

Hambone Publishing
Melbourne, Australia

Edited by Mish Phillips

Typesetting and Design by Eggplant Communications
Cover Images: Hands are healing by Rochelle Patten

First published in Australia in 2017 by Hambone Publishing

For information, contact:
The Hush Foundation
info@hush.org.au

www.hush.org.au
www.gatheringofkindness.org

ISBN 978-0-6482011-0-6

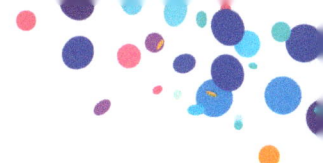

The seed of an idea

Healthcare is complex and at times stressful. It's not the only environment that feels like this, just the one that I have the most experience in. Yet I believe that the themes that run throughout healthcare - people feeling scared and vulnerable, emotions running high, stressful work situations, long and intense working hours - are seen in many other areas of society and contribute to the same problems. We are seeing recurring cultures of bullying, disrespectful behaviour, and harsh and uncaring environments.

Just when we need kindness most, it can seem hard to find.

I've been working as a doctor now since 1982, and have seen extraordinary acts of kindness. I've also seen countless examples of the converse – times when kindness was lacking and the outcome was poor. I was fortunate to meet Peter Ellyard, the Futurist, to ask his advice on running an event that would gather people together to brainstorm ways to improve healthcare culture. Peter asked me a simple question that changed my whole mindset. It wasn't "How do we reduce bullying?", which seems to be the common theme of the day. He asked me "What is the preferred future you would aim for?" My answer was "A kind health system." Kind to the patients, to the families, and to the staff who work in it.

The conversation with Peter changed the whole focus for the event we were planning.

What the event was

Together with Mary Freer, I decided to hold a new, different, and bold type of event: a Gathering of Kindness – a gathering to aim for the positive future that we want to see, and to launch a movement promoting kindness in healthcare.

We wanted to inspire and delight all those who attended by choosing an amazing, restful, and beautiful venue at Duneira in Mt Macedon, Victoria, Australia. This is a historic homestead set in extensive heritage gardens which houses a remarkable collection of art and antiquities. We wanted the event to reflect our values of treating everyone with kindness, respect, and trust. We wanted an environment that could fill people with wonder and joy.

We chose food that was fresh, delicious, and nourishing. We invited world class musician Tony Gould AM and actors led by Alan Hopgood AM, to enrich the experience and engage hearts and minds through their performances. We banned the use of powerpoint. We banned 'invited experts'.

Instead we invited a diverse group of people to share their stories with the Gathering and we called them our Storystarters.

We had a flexible program that wasn't overplanned - that made some people nervous! The format allowed us to connect, chat, and explore issues in small groups scattered through the gardens. We came back together as a large group in a huge white marquee on the tennis court to mull over issues the small group discussions had raised.

Purpose and goals

Our aim is to build a community of people interested in integrating kindness into every aspect of the healthcare system.

We wanted an atmosphere that would encourage a different dialogue amongst participants. It was necessary to acknowledge that bullying and poor behaviour exists and causes huge damage and problems. We then parked that thought, and moved towards working out ways to promote kindness, respect, and trust amongst patients, families, and healthcare staff.

Who could come

We threw the invitation out widely! We asked people to send us an expression of interest which would explain why they wanted to be part of this event, what they would bring to the event, and what they hoped to do as a result of being part of GOK.

Entries flooded in from nurses, doctors, allied health professionals, students, patients, family members, volunteers, artists, and others passionate about improving healthcare culture. The Gathering of Kindness was born and 110 people joined in.

Upon arrival, every individual received a name tag lanyard with a secret 'kindness quote' hidden inside. For some, they were a small piece of wisdom or laughter. For others, they sparked a line of thought that led to the written submissions you see in this book.

For two days in March 2016 we immersed ourselves in this glorious environment, with wonderful and fascinating company, and contemplated how many problems and frustrations in healthcare could be improved by encouraging a culture of kindness.

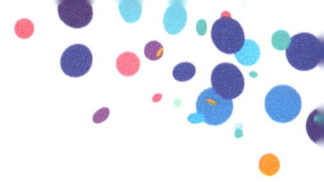

What was the result

We felt very strongly that the Gathering needed to be more than just 'a two day event' to be successful. It needed to show actionable outcomes of its own, as well as providing the encouragement for individuals to take change back into their own work environments.

To do this, we collected all the feedback using Zing technology provided by Max Dumais, on sticky notes from all participants, and through our radio interview by Rachael Kohn. We produced a summary report with a series of recommendations which was circulated to all participants, to the Victorian Department of Health, and to the Victorian Managed Insurance Agency.

We produced a short film and an ABC Radio National broadcast by Rachael Kohn on The Spirit of Things. These creations sparked many ongoing connections and conversations. We started to plan our actions for the future, including a five day GOK 2017, which will spread to many hospitals and other settings. We want people to feel confident running their own events and activities, which will build this community of kindness.

Finally, we encouraged participants to contribute to the Gathering of Kindness Anthology and over 45 people contributed to this publication. This is that book.

I encourage you to get involved in our next Gathering of Kindness in whatever way suits you.

Kind regards

Dr Catherine Crock AM
Co founder of the Gathering of Kindness

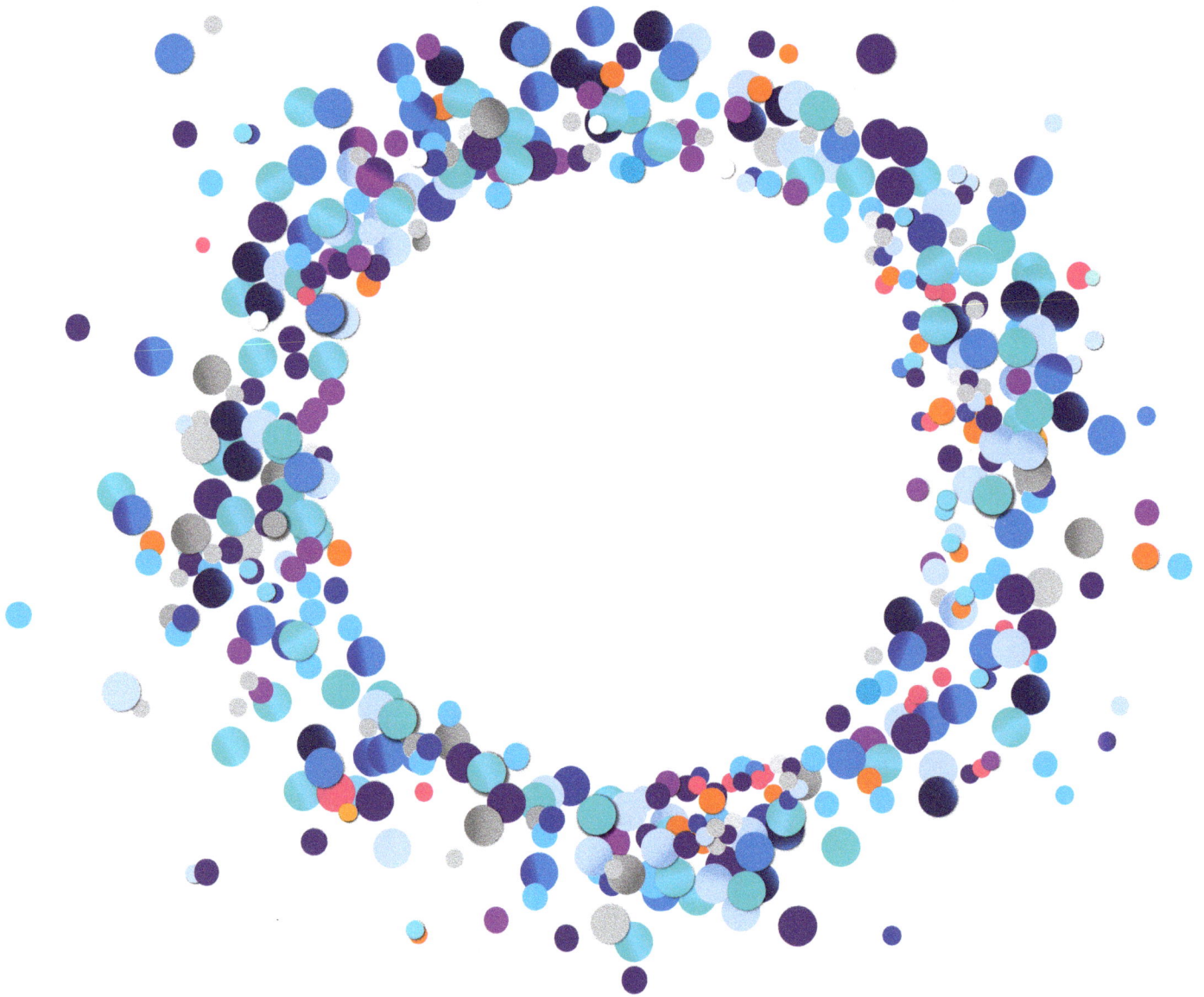

Contemplation

Understanding the Challenge

care is the context

Col Fink
Thought Leaders

The healthcare industry is, ironically, unwell.

Patients often feel like little more than statistics, especially if anything goes wrong. Doctors and staff often feel like little more than zombies, even when things go right.

Thankfully, not everyone is willing to accept the status quo.

Last week marked the occasion of the first Gathering of Kindness. It was an 'unconference' of healthcare administrators, doctors, nurses, medical students, patients, futurists, politicians, artists, musicians, and a ragtag assembly of other interested parties, including me.

The agenda was pretty straightforward. Bring together a diverse group of people and ask them to imagine what a kind healthcare industry might look like.

The fact that the question even needs to be asked when one dictionary definition of kindness is "not causing harm or damage" is somewhat frightening in itself, but the truth is that the dominant healthcare paradigm is a decidedly unkind one, which seems to treat patients as an inconvenience to be dealt with, and staff as a resource to be bled dry.

If we're to navigate our way out of this position, we need to understand how and why we got here in the first place.

As one contributor remarked; "As a profession, medicine doesn't preferentially attract psychopaths and bullies". (As a humorous aside, she added "In fact it generally attracts people who are extremely good at exams"). The unfortunate truth is that normal, caring people are indoctrinated into the pre-existing culture, eventually generating negative outcomes for themselves and the patients they're supposed to be caring for.

I don't have the time or space to write a thesis on the topic here, so while acknowledging that this is an enormously complex situation with literally millions of contributing factors, I'd like to put a finger on what I believe may be the root cause of the problem.

Healthcare has lost sight of its purpose. As Professor Don Campbell said at one of the breakout sessions I attended: "You can't treat KPI's as objectives."

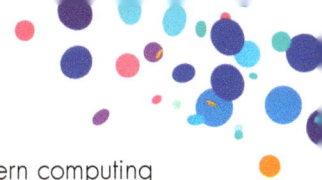

And yet, in healthcare (and many other industries), that's exactly what we do. The advent of modern computing has allowed us to develop incredible analytical power. We can measure, track, compare and contrast data points of almost limitless variety, from the finest detail right up to global trends.

Where evidence-based leadership is concerned, of course this is a great thing. Through the smart creation and monitoring of KPI's, we can minimise waste, maximise efficiency, and produce – in theory – better outcomes.

But what of those objectives that can't be easily collected, measured, and tracked as values in a database? What is the cost of suffering, and how do you measure it, anyway? What is the value of wellbeing, and what are we willing to pay for it?

We're experts on humans, but not on humanity. We live in an age where health of the body can be quantified and maximised, but health of the spirit is completely ignored. This creates excellent results in spreadsheets, and a literal living hell in the experiences of the people whose lives those spreadsheets purport to measure.

It's time to reframe healthcare. It's time to make care the context.

The Neurobiology of Kindness

Professor William T. (Billy) O'Connor
Graduate Entry Medical School, University of Limerick, Limerick Ireland.

Until recently, the task of applying what we know about the brain to the bigger question of personal human experience has been avoided by scientists. However, the emergence of the new discipline of neuroscience - the scientific study of the nervous system - is helping us to bridge this gap by providing new ways to answer such age-old questions as why does kindness exist, and why is it important? To answer these questions we firstly need to consider an important property of nerve cells (neurons) in the human brain.

The discovery of mirror neurons, a cluster of neurons in the brain that help connect us emotionally to other people, respond sympathetically towards others, and allow us to anticipate others intentions, is now believed to be the basis of human empathy. Mirror neurons were first discovered by neuroscientists in the 1990s while recording the activity of neurons in the brain. It was noticed that certain populations of neurons remain silent (observation) while others were active (imitation) when we watch others perform the same action, hence the name mirror neurons [1,2]. Scientists have extended this finding in the human brain to show that nerve activity in mirror neurons also behaves in the same way when we see another person expressing an emotion, and this nerve activity is not observed in disorders of empathy [3].

Each person is a mirror of their environment, which is then in turn mirrored by their own behaviour. This underlies the powerful phenomenon of social contagion - that information, ideas, and behaviours including kindness can spread through networks of people the way that infectious diseases do. For this reason, giving and receiving kindness can have a contagious effect. Research also shows that optimal learning takes place in an environment that is creative, inclusive, rewarding and bolstered by firm, healthy boundaries, in an environment that is kind. Even those in deep distress due to imprisonment, addiction, financial worries, and high anxiety also benefit greatly from an environment that is creative, inclusive and boundaried.

Why is kindness so important? This question can be answered in the context that every single human being is unique because we each poses a uniquely complex brain, so complex that in all of human history no two human brains can be identical. This is because the unique combination of about 100 trillion tiny brain connections (synapses) that grow and change throughout life is an ongoing work in progress from conception to death. In this way we each one of us 'evolve' as true individuals as we each make our journey through life. Kindness is the green light to keep going. If you are not open to giving and receiving kindness then you may

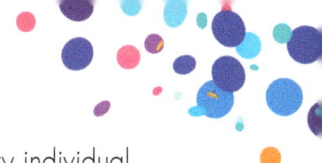

not be growing. In the same way, humankind will only evolve by making room for each and every individual to express their intellectual and spiritual evolution to the full. In this way the evolution of the human race has everything to do with being open to giving and receiving kindness.

References

1. Mirror Neurons. Society for Neuroscience (2013) http://www.brainfacts.org/brain-basics/neuroanatomy/articles/2008/mirror-neurons/
2. Kraskov A, Dancause N, Quallo MM, Shepherd S and Lemon RN. (2009) Corticospinal neurons in macaque ventral premotor cortex with mirror properties: A potential mechanism for action suppression? Neuron 64, 922-930.
3. Corradini A, Antonietti A. (2013) Mirror neurons and their function in cognitively understood empathy. Consciousness and Cognition. 22, 1152–1161.

contemplating kindness

Lynda Turnbull

It is not uncommon for people who work in the health arena to be admired by friends and family who believe they could not cope with the demands of the work. The inference can be that some people have a limitless ability to deal with the pain and trauma of other's lives. Professionals themselves may perpetuate this impression of toughness by developing strong defences and a type of immunity to suffering, with the price being a diminished capacity for kindness towards themselves and others.

Recently, over dinner with some medical and nursing friends, I raised the subjects of kindness and bullying in healthcare, as well as the potential power of the arts to engage our compassion and empathy and keep the flame of kindness alive, whether it be literature, art, movies, theatre, music. The ensuing discussion was alive with energy, disclosure, sharing and support, such as these comments:

"As a GP I am expected to get a solution. You might empathise, but you can't allow yourself to feel the true emotion, for example, hugging a patient isn't done, you are expected to be objective. In a hospital it's even more intense. You are focused on your career, advancement, finding solutions, being a good manager. You are encouraged to achieve, push the boundaries, burn yourself out. That's the ethos. We beat ourselves up if we don't achieve. Unless we realise that's what's happening to us, we get caught up in it as well and the bullying around us can be perpetuated. People who don't feel good about themselves bully."

"You can lose your own compass in a big institution and do things you wouldn't normally do. There's no time to reflect on your behaviour. You see others behaving in a particular way, so you go along, or you just see it as normal."

"Fear often underpins bullying, fear of losing power, position, prestige, reputation, face."

"When you have left nothing in the tank, for whatever reason, whether personal or professional, you have no ability to be kind. You don't care. You are more reactive to minor irritations. When kindness from others is thin on the ground, turning to the arts can be replenishing."

"If we can't be kind to ourselves, we can't be kind to others."

"The arts keep you in touch with your emotions. You have the opportunity to see, hear or do things and let them resonate. It helps you stay sane and human."

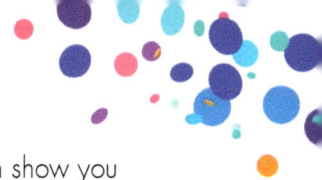

"Any of the arts allow you to engage as far as you want, but with nothing expected of you. It can show you universal truths and shared experience."

"I heard that Patti Smith, the singer songwriter, spent several days watching numerous episodes of Midsomer Murders. I get it. Sometimes it's watching drivel on TV that takes you out of a heavy space and gives you pause. I also know a psychiatrist who makes sure he watches three movies a week."

"Art animates us. Books can help us escape feelings of helplessness and despair, give us strength to carry on."

There was more, but most importantly, the conversation was genuine and heartfelt. Perhaps connecting to any of the arts could be used to trigger regular discussions of personal and professional challenges that impact or enhance the capacity for kindness. A chance to know and be true to our values and contribute to the expression of kindness towards ourselves and others that might go some way to ending the myth that we can cope with anything and everything.

Man's search for meaning

Pete Smith

"There is <u>nothing so rewarding</u> as to make people <u>realise</u> that they are <u>worthwhile</u> in this world"

- Bob Anderson

This was the quote written on the strip of paper that came with my name tag.

"How can I find my worth, my treasure
When I have no idea
What it looks like?

On a journey to seek it
That encompasses the earth
I may well trip over it on my own front lawn
On the day of my departure
Not recognising the gold
For want of the smallest spark of glitter.
Thus I search the world
Blind
Though my toe aches
From what it found in my own garden

Who can sift the glitter from the gold?"

'Man's search for Meaning' is a book that was much quoted
on the second day of the Gathering of Kindness.
I try to download it onto my **Kind**le.
But I get a message from Amazon telling me it couldn't process my request due to insufficient funds.
So much for man's search for meaning!
NOW where can I go for help?

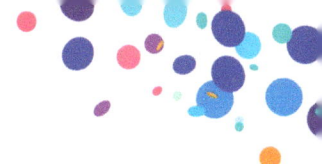

I trip over my dog on the way out the door.
I sprain my wrist.
My wrist throbs the ache of challenged self identity.
Who am I?

My response is clouded with issues from family of origin coping styles, intrinsic strengths and weaknesses, instilled virtues and values, and a cacophonic mashup of fireworks emanating from the one hundred year war between my id, ego and super-ego.

I sit on the ground holding my wrist.
The dog licks my face.

"I am who I am....." he seems to be saying, **"....Irrespective of what happens."**

I take his point.
I fell, though we **both remain the same**.

It reminds me of Milton:

"The mind is its own place
And of itself
Can make a hell of Heaven,
A heaven of Hell.
What matter where if I be still the same?"

My arm does not define me.
How I think about it defines me.

The pain dies down, an ache the only reminder of my fall
I am who I am.
A lesson from a dog.

Self actualisation will follow from seemingly random choices that lead me far from my path, though they also lead me back again to the same, now glorious, tree-lined gravel road.

Self-actualisation is its own reward.

Though I be poor, worn out, the lasting intrinsic gold will outlast all material glitter.
A treasure no man can take from me, for it dwells within me.
Take what you want, the treasure you take from me is just glitter.
Put a bullet in my head, and I will take my treasure with me,
Though I leave behind a **legacy** no gun can erase.
Maybe I know now how Munjed Al Muderis' Chief of Surgery felt when he paid the price for **not** cutting off ears.

"There is nothing so rewarding as to make people realise that they are worthwhile in this world"

My dog knows this.
He got a bone.

Who cares about bullying?

Victoria Jones

Last week I spent two days at an amazingly uplifting and inspirational healthcare event called 'A Gathering of Kindness'. This was a very unconventional gathering of visionary people ranging from nurses, doctors, surgeons and healthcare executives to academics, musicians and scientists. This was a gathering of people with a shared vision for a better, more effective healthcare system for Australia.

So what were these visionary people gathering to discuss and why do they dream of a brighter future? All is not well within healthcare, in fact there would appear to be something very, very wrong. Bullying and harassment are rife. Healthcare staff and those training to work in healthcare are suffering daily. Sadly, each year there are some who are so badly abused that they are pushed to the point of suicide.

The situation has become so acute that The Victorian Auditor General was called in to investigate the problem. Their recent report makes dismal reading

"Health sector agencies are failing to respond effectively to bullying and harassment… They are not demonstrating adequate leadership on these issues… do not understand the extent, causes or impact of bullying and harassment… do not have the fundamental, underpinning foundations of effective policies and procedures… do not adequately train their staff and managers…we found consistent shortcomings. Stronger leadership and support is urgently needed to assist health sector agencies to fulfil their responsibilities as employers, and to effectively protect their staff. The impact of poor OHS is felt not only by the affected staff, but also by the patients they are treating… Stronger management of bullying and harassment would benefit patients as well as staff… sector-wide leadership by DHHS has again been ineffective."

Why aren't we looking after the people looking after the patients?

The very people who have chosen to spend their lives dedicated to caring for others are killing themselves. Of course, there are endless policies and procedures in place, but it would seem that there are some organisations which simply hide behind these as a façade while abusing staff on a daily basis. Ignoring complaints and carrying out sham investigations, which are nothing short of cover ups and whitewashing. Those who aren't bullies themselves collude with those who are, and with this support the abuse continues. This toxic working culture has been in place in some organisations for decades, the abused have become abusers and so the rot continues. While there has been some press coverage of the issue, it generally goes on unnoticed.

So what are the costs of bullying?

There are the obvious costs – wasted time and money, loss of productivity, stress related absence, money spent on legal fees by both the employee and employer, compensation fees – the total costs are unknown millions. However, there is a far greater price being paid - the costs to lives, lives torn apart or ultimately lost for no good reason. Perhaps the sector's ongoing refusal to properly assess and address this problem is actually out of fear of facing the sheer scale of the problem and its true costs.

A hospital executive who has requested to remain anonymous stated:

"Bullying has gone on (in healthcare) for so long that it's considered normal and the millions of dollars it costs are accepted by CEOs and boards as part of the annual budget required to run a hospital."

So why isn't there a public outcry about this? This is someone else's problem, right? Wrong. This effects the healthcare we are receiving as patients. Research shows that stressed and unhappy healthcare staff are not providing the great care they can deliver. Of course they aren't. What results is substandard care for patients, patients who deserve the very best healthcare we can deliver.

There were many stories bravely shared at The Gathering of Kindness, there was much discussion about why bullies bully – insecure people, unhappy in their own lives; damaged people incapable of empathy; abuse being passed on from the top down; tall poppy syndrome; organisations afraid of individuals who they perceive as threatening their 'brand'… or is it simply a case of ineptitude?

Perhaps bullying is like an infectious disease, the abused becoming abusers. If we imagine this problem as a disease, we can see that thankfully it's not everywhere and there are stand-out organisations which are free of it. However, there are others which are riddled with it. To eradicate this disease we must identify the infected parts, cut them out completely, and only then can we begin to cure an ailing healthcare system.

Thankfully there are many who believe that we can create a brighter, better future for healthcare, free from bullying and harassment. An attendee at The Gathering of Kindness rightly said "We get the standards we accept" so maybe it's time we stopped accepting this pointless, devastating behaviour and demand more for ourselves but also for our patients. We all deserve better.

It's time for kindness

Dr Catherine Crock, AM

First published in MJA inSight on Sept 11, 2017

I started working with children with leukaemia and other cancers in 1998. On my first day on the job, I realised how extreme the environment was, where we had to restrain these children to do procedures on them.

Over the course of their cancer treatment, which lasts 2–3 years, they have repeated procedures, such as bone marrow tests and lumbar punctures. The sedation we were using was not managing their pain adequately. The children were often highly stressed and upset during the procedure, and were often sick with anxiety for days before any visit.

I was concerned about the impact of this stress on the families, so I met with a group of parents and talked with them. I asked about their experience of their child undergoing procedures. We called ourselves 'Together We Achieve'. We'd grab a plate of sandwiches and I would ask them: "What is it like when your children come in for these procedures?" And they'd say: "Actually, it's the hardest part of the cancer journey for us". But none of them had ever complained.

Blessed with the unwavering support of the visionary hospital CEO, we set out to change our small part of the health care system to a totally different environment. We started to make improvements based on feedback from the families. I became intrigued by patient and family centred care and the value we could gain from partnering with families in their care. The families knew about many aspects of the hospital system of which the health professionals were simply unaware. I realised that the expertise that the families brought to the table could improve our efficiency, reduce costs, highlight gaps in the system, improve safety and improve patient and staff satisfaction. Over a decade, the group drove a transformation so striking that children attending the hospital for a routine visit were known to complain to their parents if they didn't have a lumbar puncture scheduled.

One important aspect of this transformation arose when families talked about the challenge of being in hospital environments. "It's not somewhere you feel at ease and comfortable." The sounds and the 'look' of hospitals raise people's anxiety when they are feeling vulnerable. We talked about how we could change this for patients and families.

With the help of many of Australia's foremost composers and musicians, we set up the **Hush Foundation** to transform health care culture and environments through the arts. Since 2000, we have produced 15 albums of music that are now used across Australia to reduce stress and anxiety in health care environments.

We found that when you bring creative people into the clinical space and they experience it as artists and composers, they can see what is needed, and use their expertise to make it more calm and optimistic. It is a process that has been quite magical.

The effect of the music on patients and families is profound. But then I noticed something else. The music affected our team in the operating theatre – I could see greater respect being built between team members.

It's about feeling cared for and looked after. Musicians, composers and other artists would meet the staff and comment: "You are doing an unbelievable job. I'm so grateful for what you do, and I'd like to help". Then they made this beautiful music for us to play in our workspace. Oftentimes, the whole "feel" of the room is transformed; teamwork is visibly strengthened, and what I see as a "culture of kindness" develops. This culture has helped us to be 100% focused and engaged in our work. We all feel safe to speak up in these spaces, and we know that's important because our patients' welfare depends on it.

In 2011, playwright Alan Hopgood, AM, joined the Hush team by crafting patient and staff stories into a dramatic play called 'Hear me'. The play explores issues of communication breakdown, bullying and poor staff behaviour, patient-centred care and patient safety. Each performance is followed by a discussion forum. Qualitative analysis of 8000 audience comments and suggestions for improvement are currently being undertaken. The play has been performed over 130 times in hospitals around Australia and internationally. A second play, 'Do you know me?' has opened eyes to the challenges of Aged care.

Themes emerging from the comments show a widespread concern about a health system where bullying is common, staff often feel undervalued in their organisation, patients may not feel they are being listened to and kindness can be hard to find.

Bullying, harassment, poor staff culture and health professional stress are all topical in the literature and in the media. It is well known that these cultural issues impose high costs on health organisations through poorer staff performance, absenteeism and sick leave. Poor staff behaviour is also directly linked to worse patient outcomes.

Yet, despite these poor outcomes having been known for well over a decade, staff at all levels have been slow to accept this link. Reporting such behavioural problems is virtually impossible. As health organisations have slowly responded, the typical response has been more policies and procedures on bullying and harassment, zero tolerance statements and 'weeding out the bad apples'. These responses seem like they would help, but they are all negative and reactive. They can be ineffective and even counterproductive. And they are inconsistent with what we know about behavioural change; namely, that interventions that reinforce positive behaviour are often more effective and better accepted than those that punish undesirable behaviours.

What we need to do is change the conversation and talk instead about a kind health system and how we may get there. Because, at the moment, good as parts of it are, health care organisations are often not great places

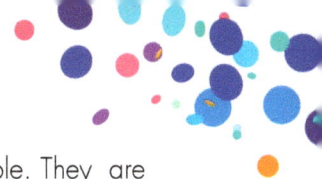

to work. They can be hard places for the patients and families when they're at their most vulnerable. They are not nearly as safe as they could be. But the answer is not to focus on the negative interactions around us. By focusing the conversation on where we want to go – towards a kind healthcare system – we can have a far greater impact. This is the mission of the second **Gathering of Kindness**, a week-long festival in 2017 that brings together people from all walks of life to continue the conversation.

Kindness does three vital things. Kindness makes best use of your team – if you are kind to those around you, then they will be there to provide support and assistance and kind behaviours in return. Kindness brings the safest environment – by fostering a culture where people aren't afraid to speak up, mistakes or risks can be dealt with openly, and before they have consequences. Lastly, kindness creates unexpected wonderful moments of joy – seeing children coming running into the waiting room, full of excitement to watch the musicians is something I will never forget.

Australian nurse ethicist Megan Jane Johnstone, who has done extensive studies on kindness and generosity in health care, has noted that the renewed emphasis on these qualities is viewed by some as "misguided" – even that "health professionals are just 'too busy to be kind'". She goes on to say that there is now a growing recognition that kindness has restorative and even curative possibilities in health care. Kindness needs to be "instated as an essential adjunct to health care interventions."

Embedding kindness in the health care system can be done. As with most major changes in health care, it helps if hospital boards are more proactive in assessing their role. It also helps if leaders have a vision of what can be achieved. But it starts with individuals – colleagues showing a level of kindness and care towards each other which will flow on to the patients and families. Let's talk about kindness performance indicators instead. Staff and patient perceptions of cultural and behavioural issues can be part of the performance assessment at all levels. It can be transformative to teams and make a big difference to the joy and meaning in our work and to the lives of the people in our care.

A smile costs nothing

Thomas Happe
12 years old

"A smile costs nothing". It's what my Gran always says to me when I'm in a bad mood and I just usually scoff at it. But now visiting the Gathering of Kindness has made me really reflect on these words. Here in the UK there is a lot in the news about how the health service is not up to scratch financially and practically. At the same time, patient satisfaction varies greatly between different trusts and hospitals. There is also a lot about mistreatment of patients in healthcare. Because of the pressure placed on doctors to work a 12 hour night shift under extreme pressure to reduce waiting times, the average doctor does not have time to give an individual service. However, giving a simple smile to a patient can make them feel more valued and positive about their care and their health, and does a smile cost anything to the doctor or nurse involved? It doesn't make them any slower and it might make the doctor feel good that they're making someone feel better. So does it really cost anything?

A connected subject is the junior doctors' strike over the new contract the UK Government has imposed. Now, I know that you are expecting me to write some piece supporting junior doctors. But I do not share the popular perception that the Government consists of a bunch of horrible people who are imposing an onerous contract. Right or wrong, they are doing what they think is best. The junior doctors, too. But kindness should be the starting point. My Gran was a nurse and she worked her way all the way up to the top of her hospital working extremely hard and had fewer staff to work with and a lot of people to care for. She made much less than the junior doctors of today. The junior doctors under their new contracts are working a few more hours a week for a lot more money in a NHS that is already in need of desperate financial assistance. Yet the bit I find most unfortunate of all is that they say they're putting patient safety first by walking out on strike, which has forced many operations to be postponed. Is this really kindness, leaving people who have waited so long and in some cases worked so hard to get ready for an operation that in reality will have to be put back many more months causing more stress and anxiety?

In my view it all comes down to a simple act of kindness and as my Gran says,

"A smile costs nothing".

What is kindness?

Hannah Wallace

"Just as elimination of poverty doesn't automatically result in prosperity and removal of disease doesn't necessarily result in wellness, addressing the issue of bullying is unlikely to provide the improvements necessary."

Dr Peter Ellyard, Gathering of Kindness March 2016

The media has recently highlighted an aspect of the healthcare culture that is disturbing. A place designed to provide care can also be a place where staff members are often not cared for and indeed at times bullied. We also know that this culture can have detrimental effects on patient care. We must ask ourselves how we can address this issue and how we can change culture. Many of our workplaces have adopted a zero tolerance of bullying policy, and whilst this is absolutely necessary, visionaries behind 'The Gathering of Kindness' Dr Catherine Crock and Mary Freer propose that we need to do more: we need to create kind cultures.

After two days of inspiring speakers and group discussion, of individual stories, of working together to understand the problems and barriers, and envisioning strategies for change, I left the conference reflecting on when I have seen kindness and what is it about those situations that have been kind.

Kindness is the renal registrar phoning back the somewhat stressed intern and immediately apologising for the delay and genuinely asking how she may be of help to the home medical team. Her tone, gentle and non-judgemental, immediately puts the junior referring doctor at ease and engages her in meaningful clinical discussion. This is kindness in action; kindness to the junior doctor who feels supported and listened to, as well as kindness to the patient, whose care is better off for a clear management plan, enabled by good communication.

Kindness is the Professor and Director of General Medicine greeting each patient with a friendly "hello" and concerned "how are you?" on the busy ward round. He does not let language become a barrier to this, ensuring he greets each patient with "hello" in their first language, modelling patient-centred communication to his team.

Kindness is the emergency consultant who stays back to help his intern finish off paperwork after what has been one of those nightmare shifts.

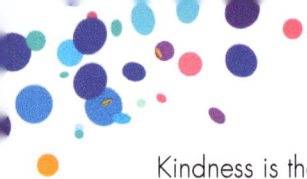

Kindness is the nurse who brings you a hot drink and some biscuits on an insanely busy cover shift.

Kindness is the elderly lady who stops to ask the junior doctor, "what are you doing here on a Friday night? You have been here since this morning." She sees the fatigue and sadness in the doctor's eyes; it has been a long week with multiple emergencies and the passing of a patient that has rattled the medical team. She genuinely thanks the doctor for her dedication and compassion, so providing the encouragement needed to finish off the mountain of paper work before going home.

Kindness is apologising for a mistake and explaining the steps that are being taken to resolve the situation.

Kindness is overcoming potential cultural, language and religious divides. It occurred in the operating theatre, where a surgeon of Islamic faith who grew up in the Middle East operated side by side with an Israeli registrar of Jewish faith, both eager to teach the female medical student of Christian faith about the operation.

What unifies these acts? It is listening, it is valuing the other human being, it is compassion, it is respect regardless of culture, language or religion, it is saying thank you, it is providing encouragement and it is acting with empathy, honesty and integrity.

Only Connect: How Stories Cultivate Kindness

Marie Ennis-O'Connor

Every word, like every person, has a story. The word "kind" is one of the oldest in the English language, dating back to the year 900. It comes from Old English "cynn", meaning "family; race, kin, sort, kind". This meaning opens up fresh possibilities for cultivating kindness. When we begin to see the universality of our human experience we can better recognise our shared kinship. Conversely, when we see another person as "not one of us", or not "our own kind", we shut down the possibility of compassion and kindness.

When asked the secret to life, novelist E. M. Forster said just two words, "Only connect". The key to deepening connection lies in sharing our stories. A single story has the power to touch us deeper than a slew of facts, figures or data points. While facts and figures engage a small area of your brain, stories engage multiple brain regions that work together to build rich emotional responses. Recent breakthroughs in neuroscience reveal that your brain is in fact hardwired to respond to story. In 2010, a group of neuroscientists at Princeton University used an fMRI machine to monitor what was going on inside the brains of both story-tellers and listeners simultaneously. They discovered that whilst the speaker was communicating to the listener, both their brains showed very similar activity across widespread areas. Their brains were effectively 'in sync' with one another, suggesting a deep connection between storyteller and listener.

"Stories seem to contain that timeless thread of human connection. This is what our brains were wired for, reaching out and interacting with others." ~ Matthew Lieberman, Social. Why Our Brains Are Wired To Connect.

We live our lives in story, we act in story, and we remember in story. Story, in the words of author Lisa Cron "is what makes us human, not just metaphorically, but literally." Story can accomplish what no other form of communication can do by offering us a chance to see life through another's eyes. A way of being in the world we may not yet have experienced. At the same time we may find echoes of our own lives. Stories are fundamental in creating common ground among diverse groups. In her essay "Re-Weaving the Community, Creating the Future", Barbara Ganley calls stories "the glue that binds hearts, souls and minds, and the force that can heal wounds between and among individuals and communities." In discovering a sense of shared commonality, we begin to see the universality of our human experience.

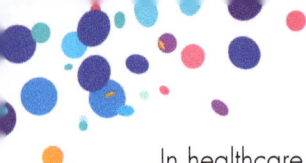

In healthcare we are surrounded by a myriad of stories – stories of pain, of hope, of loss, but also stories of healing, kindness, and caring. Each of these stories opens up fresh possibilities to nurture compassion and kindness. Within the willingness to bear witness to another's story lies the potential to offer transformative care. To enter into an experience which may live outside our direct experience requires finding a point of entry. Stories can be that point of entry, the ground we travel together in kinship; a luminous path towards kindness.

Medical kindness – more than just action

Professor Erwin Loh

Chief Medical Officer, Monash Health & Clinical Professor, Monash University

Originally published by MJA InSight

Two of the 12 apostles, Peter and John, were healing the sick during the time of the early church, and were being questioned by the religious establishment at the time about their unconventional methods. In **Acts 4:9-11**, when questioned, Peter said "we are being called to account today for an act of kindness shown to a man who was lame and are being asked how he was healed".

Even during biblical times, people were characterising healing as acts of kindness. But is healing the sick the same as showing the sick kindness? Are healers, or in our case, doctors, automatically kind? Is medicine, by definition, kind? It is worth exploring the recent literature around this concept.

Back in 1997, **Pickering wrote an article entitled Kindness, prescribed and natural, in medicine**, where the author said that to "automatically to presume it [kindness] is ever-present is quite wrong", and proposed that kindness be prescribed as part of the medical practice. So, already there is the notion that kindness is not inherent in health care, and like other treatments, it needs to be consciously prescribed and administered.

More recently, psychiatrists **Ballatt and Campling wrote an influential book titled Intelligent kindness**, which discussed the reintroduction of kindness back into the UK National Health Service and into the culture of medicine in general. This book suggests that health care used to be kind, but that somehow, over time, this kindness was lost and needs to be returned, like the proverbial prodigal son.

But how do we do this?

Let us return to our original question. Is the act of healing an act of kindness?

In his article entitled **Kindness, not compassion, in healthcare**, Faust proposed that doctors should separate the act of kindness from the feeling. He went so far as to state that doctors should "act as if they care … without taking on the stressful emotions that emanate from being compassionate or empathetic".

In other words, it is proposed that doctors can and should act kindly without needing to take on the feelings associated with being kind. This compartmentalising of feelings from action is inherently attractive for clinicians, because it seemingly offers them an avenue to shield themselves from needing to respond emotionally to the human suffering encountered as part of their daily practice. They don't have to feel kind, but they can appear to be kind, like an actor playing a role of the kind healer.

But is this acting authentic? And is this even possible? Should doctors have to divorce their actions from their feelings?

More recently, **Buetow took an alternative view in Physician kindness as sincere benevolence**, arguing that kindness by doctors should be sincere – "rather than faking it, physicians' kindness towards patients must be genuine". The author called this "physician kindness", which is considered a person-centred value that can be exercised as "sincere benevolence".

I believe that this particular frame of looking at kindness in health care is key to current medical practice. The act of kindness in healing has to come from a foundation of genuine feelings of kindness towards the patient.

I am not suggesting that clinicians need to love, or even like, their patients, but we can still be kind out of genuine feelings of benevolence towards those who are sick and infirm, as healers granted a special place in society to do so.

In a similar vein, more recently **Noel wrote an article entitled The kindness of strangers**, making the point that "after 12 years of practice, I am no longer a stranger to my patients" and that "building that trust starts with the kindness of individuals not willing to remain strangers".

Doctors must be willing to be more than just strangers to their patients. Getting to know our patients as fellow human beings, who are going through their own trials and tribulations, is the first step towards developing empathy with them, and genuinely understanding that they require our kindness.

In the words of **Wiwanitkit: "Kindness and service mind have to be the necessary requirement for any medical practitioner rather than skill and good knowledge".**

As doctors and health practitioners, let us not just act kind, let us also be kind. As doctors, we can learn the technical skills and knowledge and try to apply this to the actions of kindness, but it is important that the actions are grounded by feelings of empathy and compassion, lest they come across as artificial or forced.

The truth is, our patients can tell when we are not genuinely caring for them, and it lessens the effectiveness of the therapeutic relationship.

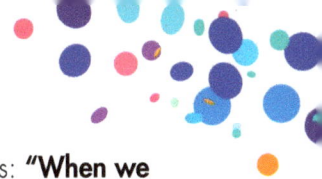

So let's get real, because we deal with real people, not just real diseases. As the Dalai Lama says: **"When we feel love and kindness toward others, it not only makes others feel loved and cared for, but it helps us also to develop inner happiness and peace."**

By being kind to others, we may very well end up being kind to ourselves.

References:

New International Version, Acts 4:9-11

Pickering, WG. Kindness, prescribed and natural, in medicine. *Journal of Medical Ethics.* 1997;23(2):116-118.

Ballet, J. & Campling, P. Intelligent Kindness: Reforming the Culture of Healthcare. The Royal College of Psychiatrists, 2011.

Faust, HS. Kindness, not compassion, in healthcare. *Cambridge Quarterly of Healthcare Ethics.* 2009 Summer;18(3):287-99.

Buetow SA. Physician kindness as sincere benevolence. CMAJ : Canadian Medical Association Journal. 2013;185(10):928.

Noel, K. A. The kindness of strangers. *Canadian Family Physician.* Jul 2015, 61 (7) 621-622.

Wiwanitkit, V. Kindness and Service Mind: Key for Quality in Primary Care. *Professor, Hainan Medical University,* P.R.China.

Robby's story

Anna McMahon

Why would I advocate for improved healthcare?

It all started after the 100 per cent preventable death of my 23-year-old son Robby.

The two day Gathering of Kindness was comprised mainly of health professionals, who were all enthusiastic in seeking to introduce a kinder method for staff to work together, ultimately creating a zero bullying, ethical, and safe work place environment.

All of those whom attended came with no expectations, yet the message was clear. Remember to be kind to others and each other. Overall the outcome was to introduce improved working environment for the health services and consequently improved experiences for the patients.

I joined the gathering of kindness, but must add I was a little apprehensive. The concept is positive, but there are so many other tangible issues that need to be addressed. I'm a professional Business System Functional Support Specialist, my job and strength is to analyse, optimise, and streamline systems, processes, and people. I believe this has given me an insight into the health system challenges.

I was there because, over the past 15 years, I have been gathering knowledge and understanding of the negative impacts and experiences of the patients and families within the health system services. I have been a very active health consumer advocate, in many different areas of health. Mainly, but not limited to the over prescribing, misuse, and abuse of prescription drugs.

Highlighting the barriers.

Robby died of asphyxiation after taking morphine prescribed to him by a doctor.

My son's preventable death has led me through a maze of dead ends and a roller coast ride across the health system, just to bring me back to where I started.

All the institutions I confronted were kind, sympathetic, and empathic, and agreed that this was a mistake by the doctors. I'm haunted every day that I failed my son, by not protecting him from the dysfunctional health system.

"If only."

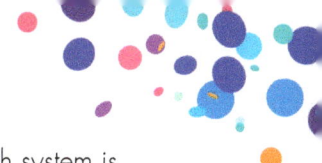

I would never have anticipated this could have happened. It was my understanding that the health system is in place to protect and care for the patients. Since the death of my son, during my advocating work, I have listened to hundreds of families and patients tell of their negative medical experiences, adverse events, and deaths. It turns out that this was many other people's understanding as well.

My journey over the past 15 years

After Robby's death, I began to ask questions.

"How did this happen to a healthy young man with his life ahead of him?"

In looking for the answer, I spoke to his new GP. He did not know crucial information about Robby, such as that he was a chronic asthmatic. Robby's previous GP was not contacted, nor was his medical file requested, before he was prescribed morphine. It was gaps like this that led me onwards.

The investigation officer at the MPBV, at the first appointment, said,

"Don't do this, don't put yourself through this. It will never be seen as of a serious nature."

Those words have been driving me for the past 15 years. What is a serious nature then? I see my son's preventable death as very serious. How can they expect me to dismiss his death? He didn't have a terminal illness. Did they think I could just accept his death? More people die from overdoses of prescription medicine in Victoria than die on the roads. Should we accept all these deaths?

I fought to bring to justice or accountability for what had happened to Robby, without success. I did not go through legal litigation as many families do, as I realised this would not fix the problem for other patients and their families. What I did instead was try to understand, and then change, the system.

The search for understanding

During the 15 years, I attended numerous court hearings and coroners court hearings of patients who died due to medical errors, or where the families believed it was a preventable death. I know that's really strange, but it was the only way I knew how to gain an understanding of the adverse events within the health system and the outcomes.

I joined numerous not for profit organisations, there to improve health outcomes for the patients and their families. I joined as a consumer representative at one of the health precincts with many hospitals and allied health. I participated in many projects to improve quality and safety, but also general improvements.

I advocated at the government and health department level, attended endless conferences, meetings, workshops, forums, and information sessions. I gave presentations, reviewed countless documents, featured in newspaper articles, Readers Digest, and appeared on television creating awareness of the importance for change to be implemented into our health system.

The gathering of kindness provided me a insight to the health professionals work place challenges, but also highlighted the compassion many have. The message was clear, they all want to work in a safe and caring environment for themselves and their peers. Plus, they wanted to be able to provide a safe and caring environment - a healthcare system of excellence with positive experiences for the patients and families.

The road to change

Over the years of advocating I have come to believe that change in health is very complex, but certainly not out of reach.

My journey has highlighted that change is not only required in the hospitals, allied health, aged care, and general practices. Change must also be realised and implemented from government agencies and health institutions through to the staff working to provide the health service.

There are hundreds of people in numerous organisations working to influence health improvements. So much energy, time, resources, funding, and good will are going into talking about the changes.

My observation and experiences has highlighted that we don't need a large budget or to introduce new governance programs. We can use the current framework to introduce change. Minor changes and improvements would be required to be implemented into the current health services, focusing on processes and procedures.

The building of good relationships between staff and effective communication between health professionals and patients could also be influenced without much effort, if these positive working process changes are implemented. Team leaders and management must enforce accountability with a positive approach rather than negative, as negative input is destructive and is not a productive or effective method to build a positive cultural change.

Learning from errors is absolutely vital. This is about taking the staff on the journey to implement change, not applying it from above. This will ensure a positive work place, and good outcomes for staff and patients.

This is what I want for my son.

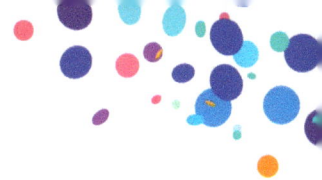

Tiny Shoes

Rosie Keely

In my mind,
The concept of kind
Is far from complex or hard.
For me it comes freely,
It's natural and easy,
There's nothing fake or façade.

I struggle within,
In the job that I'm in,
Hearing stories that tug at the heart.
For families who find,
Health care unkind,
It can simply tear them apart.

'I want to be heard,'
Isn't absurd,
When it's your child who's distressed and unwell.
Their shoes might be tiny,
Pretty coloured and shiny,
But just step in them and then you can tell.

From a human perspective,
It's not an elective,
To show compassion and care.
The components that make us,
When missing, can break us,
Of this we should be aware.

When it comes to the fore,
And we start to explore,
'Being kind' is not you defeated.
It's a choice that we make,
Do we give or we take?
Just treat others how you'd like to be treated.

Who is your ray of sun and whose foot is stomping on you?

Dr Ioana Vlad

Emergency Medicine Physician & Clinical Toxicologist
Sir Charles Gairdner Hospital

I once read a book about a rich girl treated in a big hospital in New York, whose father then donated some of his gold coins to the hospital coffers. And at the same time, in this same hospital, the junior doctor who looked after her had numerous sleepless nights and went days without proper food as his boss was a nasty bully. Despite this, the junior flourished professionally. So one of the not-so-hidden messages in the book was that you don't learn only from people who are nice to you, but that those who challenge you are just as important to make you grow. And I've been wondering about this since.

I thought about a flower that buds - what does it need to blossom? If it is stepped on over and over again it will just wilt and eventually die. But as soon as it snatches a ray of sun, it shoots its frail stalk further and further away, and eventually shows its beautiful colourful petals despite being stepped on.

My grandfather taught me to love nature, he showed me how seeds grow into plants that fruit, how chicken and puppies are born, how fruits are harvested and pigs slaughtered. My parents stepped on any idea that I had that was out of ordinary, whipping me back in line. My husband saw the seeds and nurtured them to harvest. The Lady and The Gentleman who were my uni pedagogues taught me that a smile is more important than a thousand words, and that gentleness exists despite oppression. That power has no gender and is not always expressed by swearing or physical force.

And then I moved to a country far, far away. "No, we only take the best graduates from our local schools." Just a polite "No, we don't have any jobs". Until that phone call on a late December evening when everything was dark and gloomy despite the West Australian December sunshine. "Are you still interested in that job?" It did not follow rules for sure, but changed my life forever.

One step at a time. A bit of sunshine, some more petals came out. Then some more refusals "Just because you're different." "You speak with an accent." "You should do a different speciality; you're too soft for ED." "You're wrong because you're a woman and white and younger than me"… until I glimpsed another ray of sun. "We're very lucky to have you here… have you thought about doing ED?"

34 Gathering of Kindness Anthology

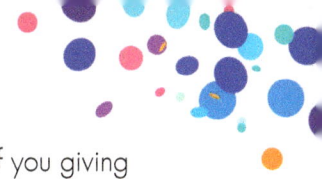

So maybe the book was right. I appreciate a smile and a thank you more in a day of "I'm sick of you giving me work to do" and of drunken and drugged swearing and spitting. Because I have a ray of sun to chase.

Now have a think. Who is your ray of sun?

And who is the foot stomping you?

And more importantly, who are you a ray of sun for?

And mind the flowers!

The Journey

Liz Ramsay

At 87 Dad was diagnosed with duodenal cancer and a year later bowel cancer. Following his second operation I accompanied him on monthly visits to his oncologist M. M. mapped out a chemotherapy program, which proved surprisingly effective after 6 cycles. Oncology visits continued and Dad enjoyed good health for the next 12 months until periodic tests revealed secondary cancers. Dad's medical regime for the next 6 months was palliative radiotherapy, an operation, and more palliative radiotherapy.

Kindness in the face of exasperation and confusion. Over the months I noticed patterns emerging in our interactions with M. He verbalised what might have been safer as an internal monologue! He mostly spoke at us. He occasionally asked questions of Dad, scarcely pausing for an answer before leaping to possible medical conditions and treatments. MGUS? Myeloma? Osteomyelitis? Bone cancer? A PET scan. More CT scans. We often came away with conflicting information about the need for further treatment, its type and urgency. And despite Dad's poor health after palliative radiotherapy, we still felt M. might push for further chemotherapy.

Such interactions and unfiltered thoughts left us confused and exasperated. After a while Dad stopped listening. I continued to take notes, hoping to make more sense of the information later, and asked questions as opportunities arose. Did we experience 'unkindness'? We certainly felt difficulty being heard, and a lack of empathy and consideration for Dad as person. Perhaps, I reflected as kindly as I could, M.'s behaviour arises from thoughtlessness rather than egotism or mean-spiritedness.

"We create ripples of energy or unease. We either create or drain energy." ~ Andy Bradley

Time for a second opinion.

Kindness takes many forms. When we met with E., she gently led Dad into a conversation that traversed his capabilities, quality of life, daily activities and mental health. She summarised Dad's medical condition, then looked at him and said "As doctors we are taught to do no harm. For you that means no more time consuming and painful interventions that have little benefit and a rising risk of harm."

Yes, E. guided us through a difficult conversation with honesty, empathy and sensitivity. But that difficult sentence was the greatest of her kindnesses. I sensed Dad's heart open as he acknowledged the short time he had left and his gratitude for a life well-lived. I too felt the space around my heart expand. I felt the transformative

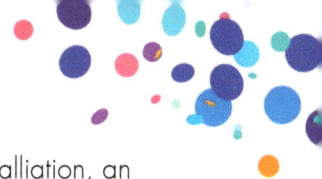

power of that kindness as the conversation and our emotional energy were directed to effective palliation, an advanced care plan and end-of-life wishes.

"People forget what you said, people will forget what you did, but people will never forget how you made them feel" ~ Maya Angelou.

Small reflection. Kindness is a choice, most available to those who befriend their own inner life. If we cultivate kindness through self-compassion, we can harvest a replenishable supply to share with others.

The Kindness of a Princess

Tanya Hendry

On 31 August 1997, Princess Diana was killed in a tragic car accident in Paris. On the other side of the world in Melbourne, Australia, an 18-year old woman was in a similar accident after her taxi driver fell asleep and had a head-on collision.

The woman was rushed to Monash Hospital and six days later, after multiple operations and time in the Intensive Care Unit, the first thing she watched on television was the funeral of the world's beloved Princess.

As this woman recovered from a broken back, leg, collarbone and ribs, ligament damage in her neck, liver and bowel lacerations and a lung contusion, her mind turned to the life of this Princess and her generous and kind spirit. Since then she has felt a special connection, and when Diana's life is celebrated in the media it reminds her not only of her own accident, but of the impact that Diana's kindness left on the world.

While an inpatient on the children's ward, this young woman experienced immense compassion from the nurses. In fact, 18 years later, she would love to see them to thank them for such kindness and understanding and for sneaking her dog onto the ward for cuddles! At the same time, this opinionated university student was completely perplexed when a group of doctors crowded her bed and the head doctor told everyone that the reason for her giant neck brace was because of severe pain. This came as a complete surprise, because she had never been asked about her pain levels and was actually feeling quite fine thanks to large doses of morphine. No one had explained to her why she needed this massive, restrictive device and when the doctors left she burst into tears about her lack of voice in this whole experience.

After a stint at rehab the young woman finished her university degree and was drawn towards working in healthcare. Her experience in hospital and rehabilitation at such a seminal age changed the course of her life. In what seemed initially accidental, but on reflection, her fate, this young woman was drawn towards the emerging profession of consumer participation in the early noughties. She is now a passionate advocate for patient and family centred care and has continued her career in this field.

So this is my story and the Gathering of Kindness reminded me of why that experience changed my life, and the connection I feel with Diana's spirit of kindness, and the reason I get out of bed every morning. When people are in hospital they are at their most vulnerable and it can be an incredibly frightening and

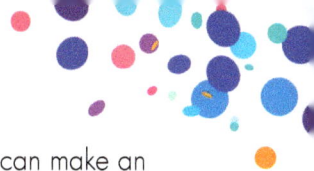

overwhelming experience. A simple act of kindness can make such a difference and believe me, can make an impact to last a lifetime.

"Carry out a random act of kindness, with no expectation of reward, safe in the knowledge that one day someone might do the same for you." ~ Princess Diana

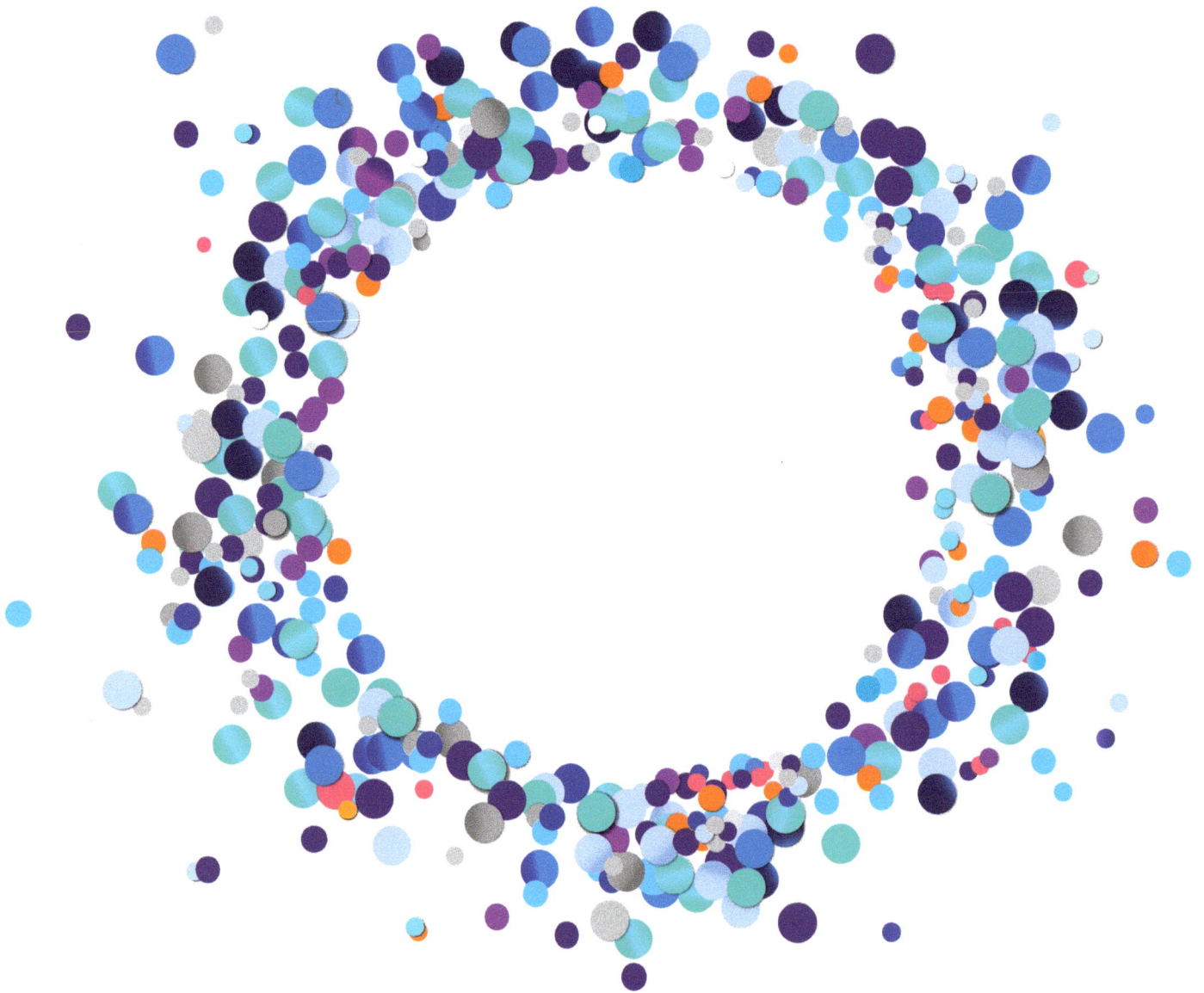

Collaboration

At the Gathering
of Kindness

At the Gathering

Lea McInerney

It's a chilly morning and mist is hanging low over Macedon's nearby mountains on the first morning of the two-day Gathering of Kindness. As I get off the train I spot three other people looking for someone. The organisers have arranged a lift for us to Duneira, a heritage house and gardens where the event will take place.

Soon we're in a car with our driver, Sharee, one of the event's many volunteers. She quickly puts us at ease and we introduce ourselves: psychologist, social worker, doctor, government policy officer, and myself, reporting for Croakey.

We're all a bit sniffy, noses cold from the sudden chill. Sharee points to a box of tissues sitting on the console. "It's colder up here in the mountains," she says. "I thought you might need these." Gratefully, we each grab one.

Two acts of kindness already and the show hasn't even started yet.

When the organisers offered Croakey a scholarship place at this very first gathering of its kind, I must admit to feeling a bit sceptical. The promo said, "We're inviting you to re-imagine a healthcare system that has kindness, trust and respect as core components." It brought to mind Gandhi's reply when someone asked him what he thought about western civilisation: "I think it would be a good idea."

I've been both inside and outside the healthcare system. In the early 1980s, I registered as a nurse and specialised in palliative care, first in hospitals, then with people in their homes. I left a clinical management role in the 1990s and became a health policy analyst, then worked in organisation development.

I've been a client of health services and have cared for family members with serious illnesses. I've encountered kindness and meanness, care and carelessness, clarity and confusion. We all want things to be better, but when your hopes have flown high then crashed to the ground a few times, you go in a little warily.

"This will be two days where we design something that doesn't yet exist. It will take courage, imagination, thoughtfulness, humour and cooperation." So the invitation promised.

The organisers, healthcare entrepreneur Mary Freer and hospital-based doctor Cath Crock, had been talking together for some time about the increasing problem of workplace bullying in healthcare. Mary is the person behind **Change Day**, a social movement that encourages people to commit to making a single change that will bring better health outcomes in their work, while Cath has been involved in developments in patient-centred care for many years and was awarded a Churchill Fellowship to study practices overseas in 2010.

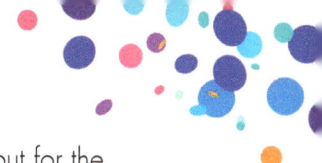

Both women were aware that bullying was likely to be a problem not only for the staff affected, but for the people they were caring for too. They talked it over with **futurist Peter Ellyard** who encouraged them to flip it on its head. Rather than try to get to the bottom of the problem, why not go straight to a preferred alternative. Not "How do we end bullying?" but "How do we create kindness?"

Around the same time, the Victorian Attorney-General's Office had been conducting an audit of data from three reviews of bullying in healthcare settings. The findings were alarming – the incidence of bullying was high, it was poorly dealt with, many workers were caught up in an escalating cycle of poor behaviour, and they had little confidence that anything could be done about it. The audit concluded that stronger leadership and sustained commitment was required from health sector leaders to make things better.

The Victorian Health Minister Jill Hennessey is now overseeing a wide-ranging strategy within her department to create a culture that supports both patient and staff safety. Last year she approached Mary to see if Change Day 2016 would do something on bullying. Mary proposed the Gathering of Kindness and the minister was supportive, offering a small grant to get things rolling. Another early supporter was the Victorian Managed Insurance Authority, which provides risk advice and insurance services for state government departments, hospitals, health centres and community services.

Mary and Cath gathered together a large group of volunteers – the budget was too small to hire an events manager – and in late March found themselves welcoming 100 people from Australia, New Zealand, Ireland and the UK to Macedon.

Sharee leads us from the car park to the booking-in table and cups of tea and coffee set up on the patio outside the historic home. People are rugged up in coats and scarves, mingling and talking, shyly with strangers, relief on their faces when they meet someone they know.

Welcoming participants

While I'm standing there warming my hands with my coffee cup, I meet the executive director of nursing (DON) of a hospital in Sydney who becomes my 'go to' person for the current state of play in hospitals. We're both about the same vintage and while I left the profession 20 years ago, she's had a varied nursing career in the UK and in several Australian states.

We dive straight into the topic. Is it worse now than in the past?

She tells me about a student nurse who recently had her first experience of giving a patient an injection. The senior nurse had given her no time to prepare and it was much more stressful than it needed to be. "She just threw me into it", the student said. If staff aren't nurtured, the executive DON says, they can't nurture patients.

I tell her I remember working with a senior nurse I'll call Beth, during my first year as a registered nurse in a hospital. Beth was always grumpy and bossy, and was the trigger for the first self-help book I ever bought, Dealing with Difficult People. I don't know if what she was doing was bullying – we didn't really use that language back then – but her behaviour wasn't kindly and it was certainly persistent.

A bell rings and it's time to make our way to the marquee on the lawns. Inside are large round tables close together, nine or ten seats at each. We settle in.

Setting the stage

Mary and Cath are up the front and welcome us all. "If you've ever been to a conference," Mary says, "forget all that now. This is an un-conference."

More on that shortly, but first Mary-Anne Thomas, the local state member for Macedon, and Parliamentary Secretary for Health and Human Services, opens the gathering, after acknowledging the Wurundjeri people. She touches on the magnitude of the challenge and quotes Rosie Batty who, when a journalist questioned whether violence against women would ever end, said that you must believe change can happen, that it's possible.

The un-conference starts off in an un-conference-like way with a performance of a play. Called **Hear Me**, it was written by Alan Hopgood in collaboration with the Australian Institute for Patient and Family Centred Care. It's now been performed over 100 times in healthcare settings in Australia and New Zealand, and seen by around 7,000 people. (If Hopgood's name rings a distant bell that's because he was Wally in Prisoner and Jack Lassiter in Neighbours.)

The play deals with the aftermath of a young woman's death in hospital after she was given the wrong medication. It's hard to watch – a heartbroken mother, an arrogant physician, a devastated junior doctor, a nurse who doesn't want to rock the boat, and a CEO trying to find a way through.

The message that comes across at the end of the play – how critical it is to properly listen to people, patients and their families in particular – will come up time and time again during the conference.

When I was in my 20s, I worked in a small country hospital for a while. I nursed an old man who had advanced cancer. He'd had treatment in the city then returned to his hometown for care. His prognosis wasn't good.

One day, as I was fixing his pillows, he said something that made me realise he didn't really understand what was wrong with him, and how serious it was. Either no one had spoken to him about his condition or, just as possibly, somebody had when he'd been in the city hospital, but he hadn't been able to take it in at the time.

In those days, in that place anyway, only doctors were allowed to talk with a patient about their diagnosis.

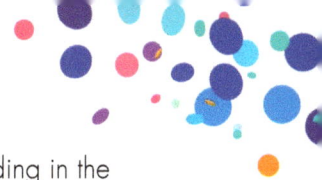

I asked the doctor if he could talk to the man, let him know what was happening. We were standing in the corridor a little way down from the man's room. The doctor said something along the lines of, "There's no point in telling him, he doesn't know what's best for himself and there's nothing that can be done anyway."

I knew it was wrong, but I didn't feel I could override the doctor's orders. The dying man, who I can still picture, was one of the reasons I headed to London to study oncology and palliative care. There had to be a more respectful way.

This is what I remembered, as I watched the play.

When it finished, Cath and the actors invited people from the floor (or, more correctly, the grass) to offer their responses.

Someone quoted a state health minister who says the experts of the health system are at both ends of the stethoscope. Another suggested that we underestimate the skills required to have difficult conversations, whether that's with a staff member or with a patient. Someone else's take on it was that, too often, the individual agendas of health professionals step in over the real purpose of what they're actually there to do.

A more personal response came from a philosopher who had recently been a patient. She was in hospital for a long time and said the nurses and doctors were fabulous and very attentive. The thing that bothered her though was the design of the hospital – the physical design as well as the systems, which she could see were often inefficient.

Because hospitals seem so concerned about safety these days, she said, patients are constantly being seen by different health professionals, and this gets tiring. She was also troubled by seeing elderly patients left on commodes for a long time, adding that obviously resources, and the lack of them, have a profound impact.

The fate of the junior doctor in the play isn't pretty – she abandons her career, a not uncommon situation – and this triggered passionate discussion about the pressures on staff, young doctors in particular, and how easy it is for their confidence to be shattered.

A doctor now in his 50s spoke about how as a junior doctor under supervision, he'd administered the wrong dose of a drug to a patient who died. He observed that mistakes at the beginning of your career tend to be through lack of experience, while mistakes by more experienced doctors often come from being too busy and missing things.

In response, another older doctor talked about how inherently unhealthy the health system is, saying that the three words he's heard over and over during his career are "Who needs sleep?" He added that we all know that people work best when they're rested and fed and comfortable. The whole profession, he was starting to think, works in a zombie state.

Someone else said it's important to recognise that health workers will get things wrong sometimes, that it's better for the system to recognise this and build a culture of learning, rather than a culture of pretending that mistakes are never made, and coming down heavily on people when they are.

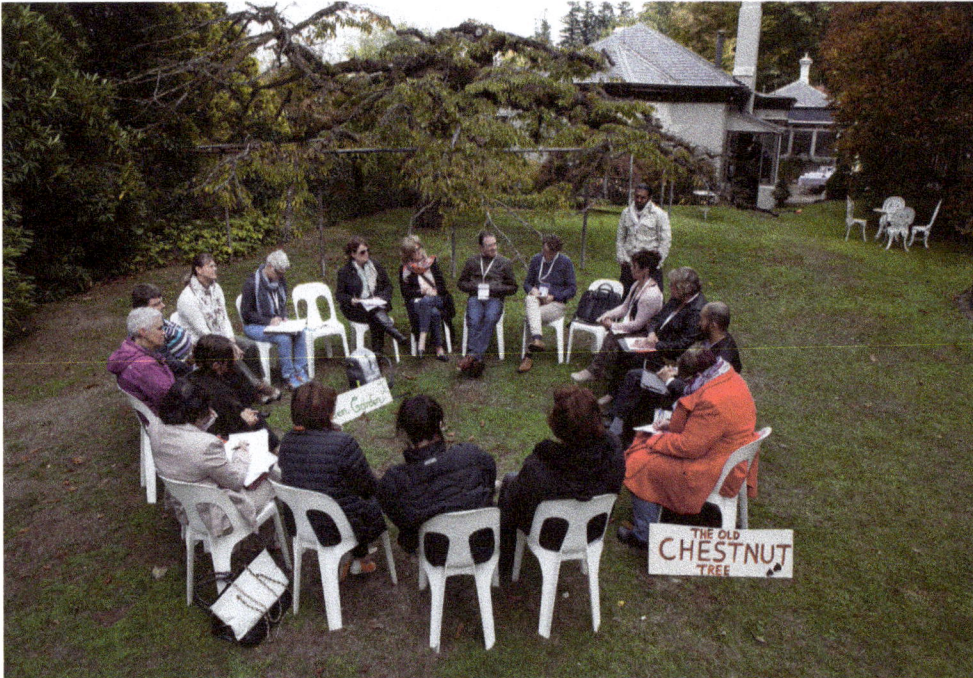

At this point I was starting to see the value of focusing on creating a positive culture of kindness, rather than trying to solve every individual problem.

Different people were canvassing causes: lack of resources, lack of leadership, inadequate management skills, poor role modelling, the way nurses and doctors interact, individualism, faulty systems, and more. It felt overwhelming. At the same time, many of the personal anecdotes were harrowing and were touching raw nerves for some. It looked like the two days might teeter between war stories and impassioned opinions about single fixes.

Perhaps sensing that, someone turned to the question of whether you can you teach kindness, to which Mary invited the philosopher to respond. She said she's not convinced you can, that it's a trait of character inculcated from a young age.

Mary then brought in Billy O'Connor, a neuroscientist. His take on it is that kindness is contagious among humans because we're a highly social species. We're born helpless, we have to be fed and cleaned by at

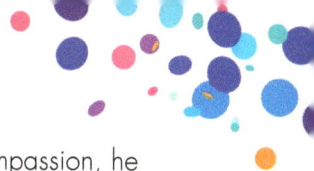

least one other human being at great cost financially and emotionally to them. If there was no compassion, he said, there'd be no next generation.

However, there's another dynamic that can undermine this, and that's often at play among professional groups – an unconscious agenda to maintain the status quo. If anything changes, he added, they lose the power they hold, and that's a big problem to have to work around.

The play and subsequent discussions helped to set the tone for this event being different to business as usual. No keynote addresses, no individual speakers, not even any PowerPoint presentations.

Instead, there were Story Starters – an artist, surgeon, physician, philosopher, musician, futurist, entrepreneur, neuroscientist, actor, lawyer, patient advocate, former patient, politician, academic, video producer – who kicked-off what were called Open Conversations.

Four or five Story Starters would kick off a session by each telling a story based on themes like "Where have you met kindness and can we increase the likelihood of that meeting?" and "Kindness in strange places". Mary or Cath would then open up the discussion to the whole gathering. The message was, if you want to join in any time, just do.

In a marquee of 100 people that could be a recipe for chaos. But from where I sat at the back, it seemed to work well, people listening intently, those doing the talking not hanging onto the microphone for too long.

In between the Story Starter sessions were Creative Clusters – small group discussions, where people met in groups of eight to ten dotted around the gardens (sunblock helpfully provided), and talked about their experiences of both bullying and kindness.

As I listened to the stories, I heard a few different angles on kindness coming through – it's contextual, it's important to consciously put people at the centre, that staff are people too, that listening is powerful. There were also lots of stories about acts of kindness that people had found very moving.

Kindness in context

What is kindness and do we all have the same picture of it in our minds?

As it turns out, probably not. Someone brought up the Christian teaching of "Do unto others as you would have done to you" and this opened up a discussion about different cultural ideas of kindness.

Sometimes there's a mismatch between the intention of the person being kind and what's actually needed by the person who is the object of a kind act. A doctor gave an example of not helping a man in a wheelchair struggle for ten minutes to get through a door, because he'd realised the man wanted to learn how to do it for himself.

Then there's the question of how do we be kind when it's a tough environment and other people aren't being kind? In response, someone quoted Abraham Lincoln: "I do not like that man. I must get to know him better."

Munjed Al Muderis, an Iraqi orthopaedic surgeon who arrived in Australia by boat 17 years ago and was held in a detention centre in the desert for a time, talked about how non-English speaking people can sometimes come across as rude. He said he went to a very good school in Iraq and was taught English, but instead of learning how to say, "May I please have a glass of water", they learned to say, "I want water." He said it took him ten years in Australia to learn to say, "May I please have the scalpel?" He added that he is married to a Russian woman and that when she speaks English she can sound abrupt.

The neuroscientist expanded on his earlier stories about kindness and compassion being central to how we've survived as a species. He talked about a recent discovery in neuroscience of 'mirror neurons', a cluster of neurons in the brain that seem to have a role in how we engage with others.

He touched on it at the gathering and later explained it like this in an email:

Each person is a mirror of their environment which is then in turn mirrored by their own behaviour. This underlies the powerful phenomenon of social contagion – that information, ideas, and behaviours including kindness can spread through networks of people the way that infectious diseases do. For this reason, giving and receiving kindness can have a contagious effect … Unfortunately, social contagion also applies to negative emotions. In this way, anger and rage and the behaviours they may generate, such as rudeness and aggression, are also socially contagious."

Prof William T O'Connor, Limerick University

People at the centre

In the discussion in the big marquee after one of the Open Conversations, Rochelle Patten, a Yorta Yorta Aboriginal Elder, told the gathering a little of her story and her people. She grew up on a river bank in regional Victoria and there were hard times, she said, "But you learn things along the way and it shapes you."

She talked about the racism that is an everyday experience for her people. Many go into hospital very sick, but come out early because they're not treated well. Recently, she had major surgery herself and experienced rudeness from staff generally, and nurses ignoring her requests for help.

She reminded the gathering of the different sorts of knowledge people have, pointing out that some people learn things in universities and become experts on different subjects, but that when they're interacting with her community, often they know "shit all" – because they haven't lived there and connected with people. Often, she said, non-Indigenous people don't understand or appreciate a person's spirit and how it's part of their story.

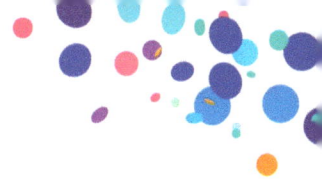

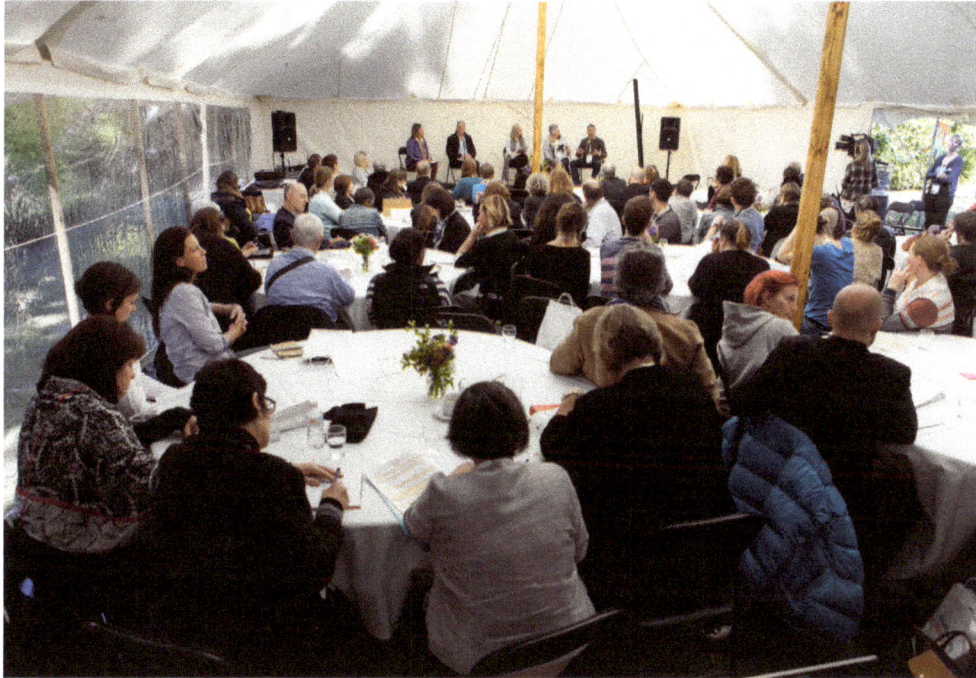

In one of the Creative Clusters, outside in the warm sunshine, the executive DON said she loves her job because of its explicit focus on patient-centred care. The CEO is totally committed to it and every decision, from senior management responsibilities through to individual patient care, is expected to be in line with it.

At every executive meeting they have a current patient story, where they look at what's going well, what could be done better, and what support staff might need for that. She visits the wards regularly and talks with the nurses, asking similar questions – what's going well, what's not, what help do they need?

Staff are constantly reminded of the behaviour expected of them. If people act in ways that aren't in line with the hospital's values, then they're called up on that. It's important, she said, to have the courage to call out inappropriate behaviour at the time it happens. People will always push boundaries, but it's important to make it within the limits of values and expected behaviour. She finished her description of her workplace saying it's a very nurturing environment, focused on both patients and staff.

Another woman who works in arts in health talked about a major art gallery where she worked for a while. The CEO held a meeting where every member of staff was present – curators, cleaners, security, everyone. The curators looked at the cleaners, a question on their faces as if to say, why are they here? The CEO began the meeting by saying everyone is critical for the work – without the security people the artworks would be stolen, without the cleaners it wouldn't be a nice place for people to visit, without the artwork, no visitors.

One of the Story Starters had breast cancer as a young woman and now regularly gives talks to healthcare workers. A question she often puts to them is, "Do you see the person behind the disease – do you see their story?" She mentioned a book called **The Wounded Storyteller** that encourages you to see an unwell person as a story with a life. She thinks we've lost that now that we have CT scans and myriad ways of testing people.

In her experience, what most people want is medical treatment and for the health professionals to 'show up', to bear witness to their suffering. She suggested that we may not be able to solve this in our current healthcare facilities, and might need to find new spaces where we can be vulnerable and find a window into our own souls. She doesn't think it's ever found in the bureaucracy or in checklists.

Staff are people too

Munjed Al Muderis, the Iraqi surgeon who was held in a detention centre, spoke about the paradox of hardship and suffering, of how it shapes you and, depending on how you respond to it, how it can make or break you.

Billy O'Connor, the neuroscientist, picked up on this and talked about the work of **Viktor Frankl**, a neurologist and psychiatrist who was a prisoner in Auschwitz during the war.

Amid the squalor and hardship, he noticed that some people retained their dignity and were consistently kind and courteous, while others seemed to give up. In time, he came to see a distinct difference between the two groups: those who remained kind had a sense of meaning or purpose for their life beyond the camp, while the others didn't.

Frankl found that while it's hard to continue to be kind in an environment where kindness is rejected, if you have a purpose, it's protective. Alluding to Harry Potter, the neuroscientist said it was like a magic cloak that protects you from bullies and catastrophes.

If you have a lot of people in workplaces who feel 'stuck' in their jobs, he said, that can affect the way they feel at work which flows onto the way they treat the people they care for. If you're doing something you love doing, you'll be happy.

You must find out what you love doing, he said, adding that humans probably shouldn't stay in the same job all their lives, as they can end up feeling trapped – although he acknowledged that family, mortgages and various other commitments mean making a move can require a lot of courage.

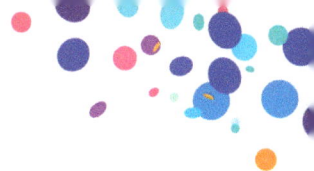

The power of listening

During morning tea on the first day I met a woman who works in a hospital and whose role is 'spiritual care', also known as pastoral care. She mentioned chart-reading versus storytelling. Chart-reading is when a health professional gleans what's going on for the patient from the chart at the end of the bed. Storytelling is what most patients would prefer – to tell their story to the people looking after them, and have them respond to that.

She's observed that many health workers, when interviewing patients or clients, have a 'checklist' approach, working their way through questions on a list. They often miss cues like a particular tone of voice or a fleeting expression that could lead to deeper, more relevant, questions. She pointed out that even just in general conversation, we're often getting our own reply ready rather than listening properly to what the other person is saying.

In between sessions, I heard a story from a young doctor about an old man he assessed in casualty one day. He suspected a particular medical condition and was running a series of clinical tests. One of them involved asking the man to smile, to see whether a bleed on the brain had affected the symmetry of his face.

Expressionless, the old man replied that he couldn't smile. "Why not?" the doctor asked. "Because I have nothing to smile about." The doctor picked up on that and asked him a deeper question. It turned out that the man's dog had died some months before and that he lived alone and had no family. He was still grieving and possibly depressed.

The doctor spent longer at the bedside and read through the man's old case-notes before making a referral to community support. Later the doctor was criticised for taking too long with patients. He knew that picking up and acting on this patient's cue, which only took another twenty minutes, would both help the man recover and prevent him getting caught up in a cycle of emergency visits, at significant cost to the healthcare system.

Acts of kindness, small and large

One of the Story Starters told a story about a senior doctor who'd had a medical emergency and nearly died in hospital. His symptoms were complicated and it took a while for a correct diagnosis to be made. Finally doctors worked out he had an internal bleed and needed emergency surgery.

Later, when he'd recovered, the doctor said the thing that brought him to tears – in a good way – was when he was about to go under the anaesthetic and realised a nurse was there beside him with her hand gently on his arm. He saw it as an expression of deep kindness and it moved him enormously. Often, it's the simple things.

The spiritual carer said members of her team make it a regular practice to keep an eye out for people in the corridors and other open areas of the hospital who might be lost.

A purpose built hospital can be an act of kindness. The politician spoke about a hospital she visited in Oslo that was built with the intention of making everyone there feel good to be a part of it. She said it's set out like a street with lots of light, and there are visual art works and also a stage where there's a performance every lunchtime. A small bridge is built out from the wards, and patients and staff can easily come out to watch.

We were given a glimpse of what that might be like when after lunch each day, pianist Tony Gould gave a short concert in the music room of the old house.

He's been closely involved with the **HUSH music project**, which involves musicians composing music specifically for people in hospital. So far there are 15 CDs, with musicians by the likes of Paul Grabowsky, Slava and Leonard Grigoryan, the Tasmanian Symphony Orchestra, Elena Kats Chernin, The Idea of North, and Lior.

Before playing, Tony talked about the care that goes into the compositions. The music's simple, but not simplistic, and not too loud or bright. There are many minor keys, but not too many. The intention is to calm people, not make them edgy.

The music room was full, standing room only, the sun shining in through the windows. As the first song finished there was a second or two of silence, people lost in their own reveries, then grateful applause.

Each piece was a gentle mix of quiet and bubbly, like water flowing along a creek. I can imagine how good it would feel to be working with it playing in the background, or if you were ill and feeling vulnerable.

Gathering up the threads

Towards the end of the first day, Mary and Cath invited everyone to start clarifying what they'd like to create out of these two days. After a wild ride of a discussion facilitated by Mary, seven specific areas emerged, among them the assumptions we make about kindness, building an evidence-base, the potential ripple effects of individuals consciously fostering small acts of kindness, and the scope for large transformational strategies.

The next day, each area was assigned its own Creative Cluster and people worked on the one they were most interested in and documented their ideas.

In another process, ten participants worked on 20 questions on kindness, recording their responses on an electronic meeting system called Zing, organised by Max Dumais, another of the gathering's volunteers. One person who took part, a consumer representative, said it was a really efficient and transparent way to collect a lot of ideas from different perspectives.

Seated around a large table, each with a keyboard in front of them, they'd listen as Max called out the questions, typing in their initial 'top-of-mind' responses. These automatically went up onto a screen above them, which was

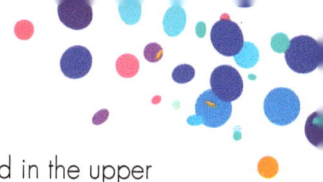

divided into two halves. In the lower half, there were ten numbered boxes, one for each person, and in the upper half, a cumulative list of everyone's ideas. As people typed their ideas in, they went into their own box, and then when they pressed 'Enter', the responses would 'zing' into the collective box. It meant that every perspective was captured and could be seen by everyone, and was available for later deeper consideration.

All the ideas from the different processes were compiled into a report.

As the two days drew to a close, Mary spoke about how we all have the capacity to help make enormous change and create a kind respectful culture in healthcare. She cautioned people to avoid creating an 'us and them' mentality towards people who use bullying behaviour, quoting Abraham Joshua Heschel who said "Few are guilty, all are responsible." This is our collective responsibility, Mary said.

Focusing on the positive, someone suggested, will need a shift from automatically saying "The system is unkind, we need to fix it" to instead saying "Let's find the kindness already there and nurture it".

Someone who works in the field of appreciative inquiry said humans tend to not notice what's working well, and we frequently slip into the negative.

The executive DON agreed, adding that throughout her career she's often experienced staff on the wards finding it difficult to identify what's going well, instead slipping quickly into all the problems that have to be 'fixed'. She has to keep refocusing them, and finds it makes a big difference when they start talking instead about the positives they can build on and use to overcome the problems.

Departure

On the train back to Melbourne at the end of the second day, one of my fellow travellers, an academic and patient advocate, put the outcomes of the gathering into context in a way that seems realistic and reasonable.

She sees it as a fledgling movement and for now it's important, she said, "to let things be little, until they start to grow for themselves."

A week later, I spoke to both Mary and Cath by phone to see how they felt it had gone, and where to next. Mary said she was particularly pleased to see such a will and appetite to think and talk about a better future – at the same time acknowledging the difficulties and the pain people have experienced in their workplaces.

She loves the "What is it I can do now?" question and where she can see it leading. Smaller gatherings are already happening in Melbourne, Sydney, and Canberra, and expanding to include people beyond those at the original gathering.

And was she disappointed by anything? Mary said she deliberately didn't allow herself to feel disappointed.

Often when you finish an event, she said, you do a post-mortem, and dwell on what you wished you'd done differently. This time, she decided to take inspiration from world famous cellist Yo-Yo Ma, who said, "It's not about proving anything. It's about sharing something."

Mary said, "We shared conversations, as respectfully, transparently and openly as possible. You always wish you achieved more, wish there was more than 24 hours in a day. But this is just the beginning."

For Cath, a highlight was seeing the effect of taking a deliberate focus on kindness. She feels it's important because you're never going to get to the bottom of bad behaviour – we've all got a bad story to tell and it's not necessarily helpful to keep going over them.

She and Mary had talked about whether to put on the play because of the negativity in it, but decided it was important to let people see, experience and feel those difficult aspects and acknowledge them, then begin to move on to a preferred alternative.

They knew it could be very Pollyanniaish to just say, "Let's all be nice". "You've got to acknowledge that other stuff," Cath said, "beause it is really bad. But rather than blaming the department or CEO or manager above you, we need to move beyond blame and all make this shift, bit by bit, into a big movement."

Mary and Cath will put their heads together in the coming weeks and be in touch with the group through different media. "There'll be another conversation and we don't know what it is yet," Mary said. She's confident something incredible will happen. "We're up for the surprise."

In the meantime, I'll leave the last word for now with the executive DON: "It's time to see kindness as a strength."

Full article at: **https://croakey.org/join-the-gathering-of-kindness-in-creating-a-better-health-system-a-recommended-longread/**

A sense of power

Alan Hopgood AM
Actor/Playwright - "Hear Me"

When I was a young evangelical, I would attend Conventions, where, even when considered retrospectively with understandable cynicism, I remember a strong feeling of a united force for good. Of wanting to put the wrongs of the world to right, even if using the simplistic recipe of religious fundamentalism.

It was powerful.

It was another 70 years before I would feel the same sense of power captured in one place - The Gathering of Kindness – which seemed, initially, to me, rather ethereal.

I salute the vision of Cath Crock and Mary Freer, who, themselves, admitted they didn't know what would happen, bringing together such a powerful group of people in the belief that something would have to happen – and it did – and restored my belief that there was still good - and kindness - in this battered world.

And as each story-teller spoke, one after the other, so insightful, so inspirational, I almost reverted to the old days and stood to my feet and yelled - "Amen!"

– but I didn't.

Kindness Vectors

Michael Axtens

I've just returned from the amazing Gathering of Kindness. Thanks so much Mary Freer, Catherine Crock, countless volunteers, and countless contributors who gave so generously in so many ways!

I've just opened a secret message in my lanyard pouch too. "A single act of kindness throws out roots in all directions and the roots spring up and make new trees" - Amelia Earhart. Thanks heaps Michelle Phillips... your acts of kindness are many!

I'm writing this as a tribute to a fresh community of people who managed to spend an amazing two days together and share so much warmth, generosity, compassion, kindness, and love.

I am thankful for the wisdom from Rochelle, a Yorta Yorta elder who said to me at one point "Too much opinion!" This was an incredible gift as it encompassed, in three words, a personal struggle I have. What is this article, for example, if it's not "Too much opinion?" and how do I rectify that? How much is "Too little opinion?" and how can I do 'kind opining'?

The Gathering of Kindness - So many different experiences brought together! How do we meet and minimalise the effects of accidental practices of invisibling, overentitlement, opining, and all those things common to Western Culture?

Thanks to Kate and others who sat silently, gently modelling of acts of patience, forgiveness, silent deep appreciative listening, and humility in spite of the possible or real disempowerment performed by those of us with 'entitlement to speak'. I'd love to have sharing of 'What kindness is to me' at the next gathering, perhaps with a 'deep listening' session. I wish I had been more silent and observant of kindness in action, but I spent a lot of time in relationship with enthusiasm, distracted from communing with and learning from the wise. I did do my best to align my goodwill with my actions.

I was amazed by the lack of conflict, or even when there was dissent, the respect demonstrated by those present. I was surprised by my own reactions to the rare statements that unintentionally risked 'othering'- diagnosing or labelling others, or trivialising their experiences.

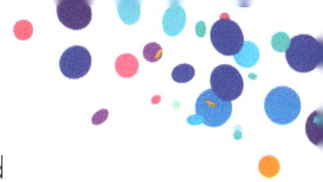

Examples were Captain Cook's 'kindness' which when pointed out, was thankfully acknowledged apologetically by the speaker (Billy) as not representative of the indigenous experience of said Captain. How many times have I chosen an example with less than universal appeal when illustrating a point? When we talk about kindness, how can we better consider to whom and at whose expense?

I also struggled with the relationship between silence and politeness with kindness. There's an interesting article titled 'Angry rebels are more compassionate than nice people' that explores this issue - thanks Gnat Atherden for bringing it to my attention. It has me still questioning "When is it kinder to be silent, and when is it kinder to speak out?"

I was also challenged by the idea that "Some people are programmed with a relative incapacity for kindness", not because I don't believe it to some extent, but because, to paraphrase Michael White, I haven't found it to be a particularly useful thought from which to proceed. If I believe low kindness is predetermined, and this deterministic thought diminishes my hope for change of that individual, then how does that not limit my options for interacting with him or her? I prefer the hopeful commitment; "I will learn from this person, engage responsibly, and find areas where kindness can be encouraged and nurtured", relegating "kindness is preset" to the background.

And what of the thought:

"Because I'm well intentioned and reflective, my acts will be intrinsically kind, as long as I'm in touch with my intentions and I'm reflective, before I act."

How do I reintegrate the truths in this, when this belief didn't work consistently well enough for me in the past? When my 'kind acts' weren't experienced as such, I integrated "to check on one's actions is essential." How can I seek feedback from the recipient without it being seen as a conditional act of 'self gratification'? Maybe I'm too attached to the checking and I need to dust off 'good intentions guarantee the actions' a bit!

Sorry too, Billy, that I failed to empathise with your enthusiasm about mirror neurons, because I was unkindly judging this as "Science colonising ancient knowledges"! How dare I use deconstructionism in such an unkind way! As a consequence, I ironically missed this opportunity for the warm/fuzzy/oxytocin laden experience of mirroring Billy's enthusiasm. To miss this was a no-no for me at a Kindness Gathering!

The whole weekend was so positive and kind, it overshadowed these challenges with the hugeness of experience of connectedness, common goals, we-ness, commitment, love, and authentic generosity. This was/ is a very special gathering, and in its steadfastness to propagate, I'm sure the inspiration, thoughts, hopes, and commitments it has created will infectiously grow in most (dare I say all?) who attended.

It really was kindness in action. I was elevated to tears by Rochelle's gift to Cathy Crock, moved profoundly by Munjed and I was silently appreciative of the love in action by so many people. Mary Freer and Cathy Crock, thank you so much for starting this! In loving appreciation of all "kindness vectors" (OMG that seems a bit like "velociraptors"!),

Thankyou!

References:

'Angry rebels are more compassionate than nice people' https://engagedbuddhism.net/2015/08/05/angry-rebels-are-more-compassionate-than-nice-people/

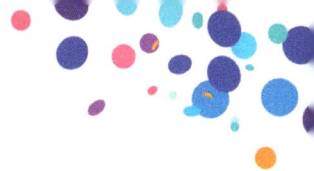

Convictions

Kate Eve
Eastern Health Manager
Spiritual Care

I feel that long ago someone may have shared with me from their wisdom, saying: "The most important convictions are not those we hold but those that hold us." For this I am grateful and now I wonder... perhaps those among us who are kindest are held by the conviction that others are worthy of love.

The getting of wisdom

Sharee Johnson
Psychologist, Executive Coach

Being at the Gathering of Kindness was not so much about learning new information. It felt more like the getting of wisdom.

The Gathering of Kindness was a big event based on a small idea, a simple idea… be kind. Or was it a small event, a moment in time, capturing the grandest idea of all?

As a member of the planning group I had thought about the Gathering of Kindness a lot. I was on the planning group because I had been thinking about it for a long time before that! Though, not as long as Cath had been - she had been thinking about it, and acting on it, a LOT! If Cath could do what she had done, imagine what 100 people all joining forces could achieve. Even the idea of 100 like-minded souls working together to bring more kindness to health was inspiring. I couldn't wait to listen and learn.

Now three weeks later I find myself remembering Marie Innes-O'Connor showing me what enthusiasm looks like as she overflowed with excitement, words tumbling from her with such eloquence. The message that still lives with me: when is the right time to witness another's pain? How do we make the new spaces where we can go beyond the words? Kindness is not to be reduced to a box we can tick. I understand this as: kindness is present, in the here and now… mind, body and soul kind of presence.

Billy O'Connor prompted me to rethink what we know about mirror neurons. Medicine is always looking for the science, the evidence base. Here is a way for me, a psychologist, to help people join the dots. What if I could have a direct impact, scientifically speaking, on your brain, structurally and functionally, simply by smiling at you? Touching your arm? Sitting down for just a minute or two? Thank you Billy for crystalizing this for me. The Gathering of Kindness did this over and over again, helped me see and feel new ways to share the information.

Being at the Gathering of Kindness felt more like the getting of wisdom than learning new information. It is affecting my thoughts, my actions and my feelings. I hope I am engaging in lots of really useful kindness that can be mirrored everywhere. Kate reminded us to listen. I was privileged as a volunteer to have the chance to listen and observe and I noticed lots about how people told their stories. In particular in this space the stories were ones of forward looking, not problem solving. Peter captured this beautifully with his phrase 'Purposeful

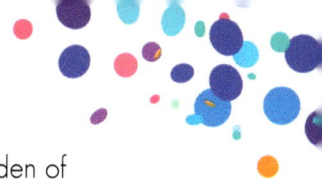

future maker'. There was a different level of consciousness there in the middle of that graceful garden of Duneira. I left with big ideas and small ideas, a big soulful community and a renewed, vibrant commitment to be kind.

"Be kind whenever possible. It is always possible." ~ Dalai Lama XIV

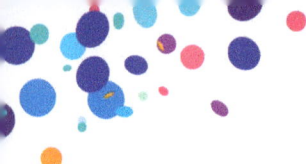

Kindness

Eve Wilson

Kindness
How can one word carry so much intention?
How can one word possibly hold such depth, emotion, community and goodwill?
Kind-ness
Kin-dness
Even broken into two to share the load – it makes no sense
Love and compassion wells from the deepest depths
Somatic and indefinable
Kindness turns me inside out, upside down, all around
How deeply can I surrender, integrate and live from this place?
Kindness

The Gathering of Kindness

Grey Searle

Clinical Psychologist
Western Health

When I saw the notice for a gathering of people interested in how kindness can be promoted in the health system, I was inspired and keen to meet such people Servant Leadership has been a cornerstone of my own practice in healthServant leadership embraces 5 key concepts – trust ,respect ,understanding ,communication and kindnessAnd gosh here was a gathering of people attending to kindness.

I came together with 99 other kindliness beacons and left after two days with a strong hold on a belief that change is possible and there is a way forward to improve the interpersonal care we provide when we are tending to the sickWe may be very efficient and skilled in our medical care, but this is only one factor in contributing to a patient leaving our care feeling valued through everyone doing their best for themYet patients post story after story telling of experiences that are quite the opposite of this.

Imagine the culture and emotional climate of a ward if above the entrance was 'Welcome to the ward of kindness'Such a ward might have taken workshops living out the Protective Behaviours themes – 'We all have the right to feel safe at all times' ,and 'No matter how awful something is, we can always talk about it with someone'Imagine a ward where all staff signed a statement of commitments :I heard about senior staff at the Royal Children's Hospital doing such a thing ,why couldn't the same process occur for ward staff ?For example ;'Our commitment is that we will treat each other with respect ,listen to the needs and concerns of the people in our care and do our best to meet them ,we will encourage the involvement of your family and loved ones in your care if that is your wish'… to name just some possible statements of commitment.

I agree wholeheartedly with Penelope Campling, who promoted the idea of a benign caring culture that would make outbreaks of cruel neglect and abuse of patients less likelyShe argues that creating and sustaining such a culture is dependent on being able to confidently articulate the positive values that should define healthcare culture through a conscious focus on the concept of "intelligent kindness". (1 ,p1)

Another valuable idea arising from the Gathering of Kindness was the idea of preserving a person's dignityThis concept eventually led me to the Nursing Times Ethical &Compassionate Nursing Supplement 2011 A notable conclusion :Genuine compassionate care is not a quantifiable skill ,an assumed technique or an emotion or feeling – it is the humane quality of kindness. (2 ,p5)

Having a professional approach doesn't mean assuming your patient-client trusts you unreservedly, but assuming instead that being professional is earning their trustl move forward charged with the mission of inspiring ,nurturing ,encouraging ,protecting and teaching kindliness in the care of patients and ourselves.

In 1878 Catherine Wood ,the lady superintendent of the Hospital for Sick Children ,Great Ormond Street ,wrote :"Gentleness of the heart will teach gentleness to the hand and to the mannersl can give no better rule than to put yourself in your patient's place." (2 ,p5)

If a patient-client of mine complaints of heartless care, I will encourage them to declare the following if they experience it again :"I am finding your attitude towards me unkind ,I wonder have you ever been a patient yourself ?"

References

1   Campling P. "Reforming the culture of healthcare: the case for intelligent kindness". BJPsych Bulletin, 2015, 39, 1-5

2   Middleton J. (Ed) Nursing Times: Ethical and Compassionate Nursing Supplement 2011

Not a Cross Word at the GoK!

Pete Smith

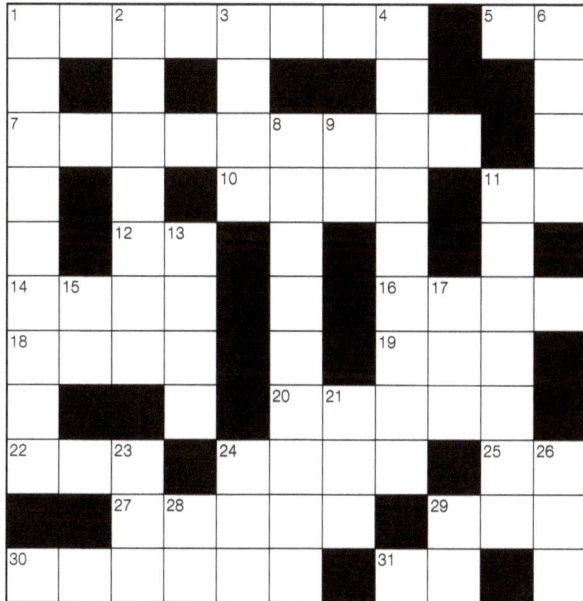

Not a Cross Word at the GoK!

Across

1 Gathering of....

5 Cogito ergo.....something

7 A Great Rushin' Queen of Kindness

10 When push comes to shove. For starters, does everything not tally?

11 Moi, moi-self and eye possess a pronoun

12 That is!

14 Hush! Someone's playing on the piano!

16 Create a lasting impression: set kindness in stone

18 This cherub is almost an angel. She never quite gets

20 A lot of work to give something worthwhile the edge, but even coffee doesn't happen without this

22 "We, ___ People of Kindness!!!!!!"

24 I have a one sided view of Kindness: Judgement can buy us.

25 Upon

27 Piano at its best

29 One-one was a racehorse. Two-two was one too. How many races did One-One win?

30 Mr Ellyard is down the road at 2050

31 A Member of the Order of

Down

1 Firing up a revolution, a boot at the commencement

2 Zero the Hero. The best things start from here. Mu.

3 I used to want, but now I knead

4 I make, I create, a bit like plastic.

6 Freer at first

8 As we go Towards 2050, pretend the future is better as the confusing migraine eases.

9 Not out!

11 A Mount forms the centre for a Gathering of Kindness

13 Windows of the soul? Aye aye, aye aye aye.

15 Go forth, carry ___

17 On the decimal scale, you are perfect!

21 Far out, man! Lets be radical. Ionise kindness and make it supercool!

23 Initially, Exceptionally Great Thinking takes place in a tent!

24 Black sheep sound like they want a drink

26 The One, New and prototypical

28 Be honest. Is this day OK for you?

29 Recitation of the Profound

Expectations – A view from the other side

Rhiannon Jones QC

Successful outcomes in medical intervention cannot be guaranteed. So what expectations are the protagonists in the medical treatment scenario entitled to have? By this, I am referring to both the patient and the clinician.

The patient should be able to expect that that the clinician has come to work fit to work and ready to try to do their best for the patient. The patient can also reasonably hope that their problems are listened to properly, not hurriedly. This does not just mean making a list of their symptoms, but it means taking on board the impact that these symptoms are having on the patient's life and those close by. Listening in this broad sense is clearly vital to best enable the clinician to make the correct diagnosis , to help the patient reach the decision about treatment options which best suits their circumstances, and to obtain effective consent to treatment. The connection formed during careful listening is vital to a constructive relationship between patient and clinician.

The patient is also entitled to be treated with dignity, sensitivity and kindness. This involves thoughtfulness, but no cost. It requires practice and is not always easy to implement in highly pressured situations, when time is often of the essence. Such gestures form lasting impressions on patients and their families even when the final outcome is unhappy. Accounts of treatment often include comments such as "I'll never forget the doctor/nurse who took the trouble to ………"

The treating clinicians need to be mindful of the fact that although they experience similar scenarios on a daily basis as part of their jobs, the patient's experience will be far from mundane or an every day occurrence, and will probably be causing them anxiety. So far as the treatment is concerned, the patient is entitled to expect that the clinician will only undertake treatment within their capability and do so to the best of their ability. At the end of treatment, whatever the outcome, the patient is entitled to a discussion of what went wrong, what went right, what the future is likely to hold, and their options.

So if that is all that the patient can expect, what can the clinician expect? They can expect to be shown respect, and to be treated courteously. The clinician can expect to be shown some understanding when they are torn in many directions due to lack of staff, lack of beds and lack of support, yet are still doing their best. They can expect to receive some understanding that they are not a miracle worker.

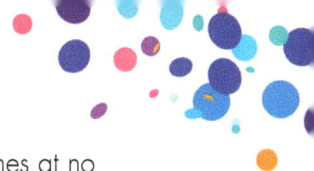

Reciprocity of kindness between patients, their families, and their clinicians would improve outcomes at no cost. Our mirror neurone systems mean that we innately contain the catalysts for good interactions if we start off consciously on the right footing.

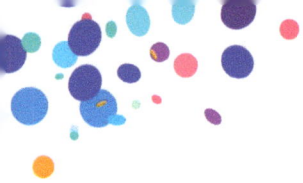

Kinship

Noni Bourke

Kinship at its core

Investment in each other

Nurture and develop, don't tear down

Do an act of kindness, help one person smile

No act of kindness, however small, is ever wasted

Empathy - walk in the shoes of another

Support each other, support those we care for

Show someone you care

To talk about kindness is also to talk about pain

Alexandra Armstrong

I have had the great privilege to bear witness to many patient stories, both as a clinician and later working in the patient experience field. I have always been struck by the small acts of human kindness that have resonated so deeply with patients and families, that they have been able to recount years or decades after they have happened. The compassion demonstrated by healthcare professionals in a patient's time of need can have such a profound impact on them. I often wonder if staff have even the slightest idea of how much that act, that word or that smile has helped a patient or their family. Every encounter offers an opportunity to leave a lasting mark, it's a great power that I believe many of us take for granted, or perhaps aren't even aware that we hold.

Likewise, where compassion and kindness are absent, we have the power to cause great pain, distress and anxiety, even if it is not our intention. I'm a firm believer that the majority of people who work in health are not intent on causing emotional harm to their patients or families, but we know that this happens, every day. Sometimes we hear about it through a formal complaint, sometimes we will never hear that person's story and will never have the chance to apologise for how they were made to feel. I wonder how many patients and families are unable to recover, heal or move forward because of an experience they had in healthcare where they felt that they were not treated with kindness, compassion or respect. I wonder what toll this has taken on them.

What I was not expecting at the Gathering was to bear witness to the pain and suffering of those in the room - of staff working in health who, like the patients and families I have met, were carrying painful memories. I wondered if anyone had ever apologised to them, I wondered if this would have helped them recover, heal or move forward, I wondered how many good people our industry has lost because of unkindness.

The Gathering was a place of positive thinking, of optimism, of enthusiasm and excitement, but it was also a place where people opened up and shared their pain, their sadness and their frustration. My approach to my position has been to immerse myself in the stories of our patients and families, after the Gathering, I've realised the importance of listening to everyone's stories. The link between how we treat each other and how we treat patients, families and carers is now, in my mind, stronger than ever. I want to be part of a movement that changes the industry for the better, to create a kinder future for everyone in health.

What's going on around healthcare?

Nathalie Martinek PhD
Conflict Solutions

Leading up to the Gathering of Kindness, I'd been studying a sacred Kabbalistic text written by Rabbi Moshe Cordovero in the 16th century. This text covers the virtues, and provides instruction on how to behave when we're faced with tricky behaviour from others. According to this Rabbi, it's not kindness that is the most important to assure a peaceful co-existence, it's humility. Humility contains the entire spectrum of virtues, including kindness, which would suggest that being humble also means that we're being kind, compassionate, understanding, and tolerant. It also means possessing a reverence about life and those we're here to serve through our professions and vocations. Humility itself is humble in that it doesn't need to attract attention to its actions, as it goes about its business leaving its impression on those who encountered it. Humility knows its limitations and knows its strengths and can feel satisfied with being of assistance, sharing its gifts wherever it can without any fanfare, need for acknowledgement, or external validation.

It also occurred to me during the GoK that no one mentioned the silent partners of mainstream healthcare. What about those who receive the patients whose journeys with their medical doctors, nurses, psychologists and social workers needed to end? Maybe they were unsatisfied with their care, or their deeper needs were unmet through the transactional nature of health practice. The multi-billion dollar industry and communities of practice that sit outside convention, but are no less interested in patient care, safety and healing. These practitioners work to fill in the gaps that formed from the shift from supporting healing to operational values and economics of healthcare. What about patient values? Spiritual and religious beliefs? Focus on healing from within using mental techniques, traditional healing methods and spiritual principles that bring peace, restore hope, and strengthen faith? Are these virtues not the actual healers?

Maybe we need to be curious about the complementary practices and approaches that many of mainstream healthcare's patients and families are engaging with and benefiting from. What are they doing that is so effective that we're not? How are they demonstrating kindness and humility and respect? Humility is acknowledging our own limits of knowledge, expertise, and experience and having the ability to say to a patient and their family, "I don't know" and "This is your opportunity to learn about what else is out there that can support your vision."

Perhaps the answers to healing and transforming the healthcare system can emerge through correcting and healing the effects of countless acts of unkindness we've experienced, witnessed, and might even have inflicted

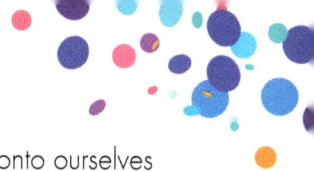

on ourselves. We can start by showing ourselves kindness. Maybe learning how to turn kindness onto ourselves means that we become kindness, so that it's the imprint we leave with others long after our interaction has ceased. That wherever there is mastery in self-kindness, or kindness embodied, that person, team or community form a field that can repel unkindness from the vicinity. Let's build a culture from kindness embodied so that the trek to humility is within our collective grasp.

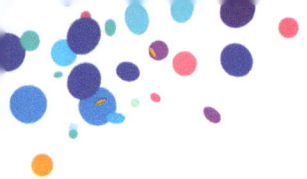

Kind-Tree

Sandy Ashton

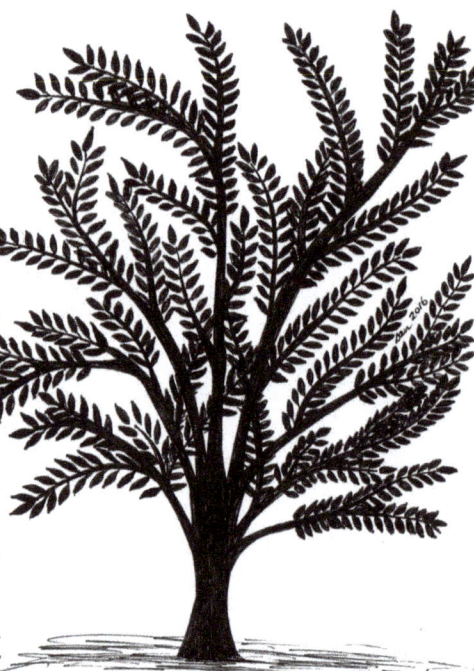

What does Kindness mean to me?

Marianne Hunter

This is a question repeatedly thrown up at the Gathering of Kindness – and people are passionate about it. Did we find the answer at the end of the two days? Well yes, I think we did. But not in the way you might imagine.

I'm personally inclined to believe that the combination of context and perception will always present a conundrum for us human folk. For example, what is considered 'kind' in one culture can be interpreted as quite the opposite in another – just look at the research from Fons Trompenaars! Plus, so long as we allow each other to experience the full gamut of emotion including anger, sadness, fear... and not just strive for the trappings of happiness, then it must be deduced that moments of bad behaviour, and even bad intent, will prevail. But that is just my opinion. There were many other views at the table – and clusters of not more than 3-4 could be seen to align in their views.

Some felt that kindness was a definable set of behaviours and intentions. Others were somewhere in between. Some felt that we should progress the cause from a place of pure positivity. Whereas others, who had been deeply impacted by bullying behaviour, clearly needed to explore their experience and put a name to it as part of their healing process – not unlike what we have experienced in recent Royal Commissions. And this exploration and debate went on over two days.

So what was the answer I referred to? It just sounds like another talk fest, I hear you say. No, it wasn't. For me the answer was that we are all unique, sensing, perceiving individuals with diverse, rich cultural and experiential lives. And we will never perceive neither kindness nor bullying in the same way.

Successful Fortune 500 companies don't succeed, adapt and grow in this ever evolving environment by accident. Something most of them have in common is that they do not simply pay lip service to Diversity - they live it and breathe it in their global companies. Our public sector organisations need to take a leaf out of their book.

I would argue that many of our health systems still have a majority of white, middle aged, and mainly males serving as Ministers, Board and Executive members. This type of Governance simply cannot cater to the needs of our very real, multi-cultural, multi-aged and gender diverse society. I can't tell you how many 'Strategic meetings' I have attended about Aboriginal health, for example, where there wasn't a single Aboriginal or Torres Strait Islander person in attendance. It made me wonder what our early Feminists would have thought about an all-male committee meeting about women's rights?!

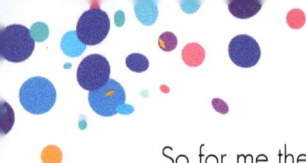

So for me the answer is that we need to start with an Aboriginal person on every Board and Executive group. Not just because otherwise positive health outcomes will continue to evade us, but because the rich culture of our First Australians has much to teach us about relationships and kindness – as opposed to our continued focus on timeframes and outcomes alone. Once this is in place, then let's continue to build real diversity into our workforce. That's when kindness will start to grow, because we will be constantly learning from one another, reduce our fear of the unknown, and perhaps even hold back on our assumptions and listen to each other.

My reflections on GoK

Geoff Coombe

The quote I received along with my name tag was: "A person who is nice to you but rude to the waiter, is not a nice person."

This is very true and relates to kindness. Kindness must be demonstrated to everybody to be kindness, otherwise it is just another tool for some people to use to portray an image of themselves.

Everyone has the potential for kindness and I think it comes from within each of us.

So, my reflection on the GoK.

For some reason when I was reflecting on GoK, The Woodstock music and art fair of 1969 came to mind. Woodstock was a representative of the hippie counter culture reacting against the societal constraints of the 1950's and the extreme unkindness of the Vietnam War. (Unkindness is hardly a strong enough word to describe war, but I will use it for the purposes of this reflection.)

After the event Woodstock gained the moniker 'Three days of peace, love and music'. Due to unforeseen circumstances, Woodstock turned into a free event over three days attended by... 500,000 people! Organisers were expecting 50,000. Obviously, all resources were woefully inadequate. To add to the problems, on the second day there was a deluge, which turned the site into an enormous quagmire. Despite these hardships, everyone demonstrated extreme kindness to each other. People were born at Woodstock, possibly three people died, and there were drug issues. Sounds like a hospital or community emergency. Health professionals volunteered their services, because they believed in what the people were trying to achieve - living in peace and harmony with their neighbours.

So, how is this relevant to GoK? The GoK could be viewed as two days of peace, love and music. I think GoK came about partly as a reaction to the current unkindness which is prevalent in the medical system, health services generally, and even in the wider community. GoK certainly did not experience the hardships people experienced at Woodstock. However, the incredible people who volunteered at and attended GoK are all looking for new ways to work and live in a 'kindness' environment. There were so many amazing discussions and ideas put forward. The tent was constantly full of energy and enthusiasm. It was wonderful to see so many younger people attending who are just starting in their medical careers. Just as the people attending Woodstock were looking for a new way for society, so the people attending GoK are keen to create a new way, particularly in the broader health systems. There was a lot of support for each other demonstrated at GoK, perhaps reflecting the lovely words of Lennon and McCartney, sung so amazingly by Joe Cocker at Woodstock "I get by with a little help from me friends".

P.S. For those of you who are interested, amazing performances at Woodstock helped launch and consolidate the careers of Joe Cocker, Santana, The Who and Ten Years After. Alright, so I love the rock music of the 70's.

Creation

Changing the future

Gathering of Kindness

Lara Giddings MP
Former Premier and Health Minister in the Tasmanian Government

To be kind takes not a moment; to undo the damage of those who have been unkind can take a lifetime.

We all live busy, stressful lives in this modern era trying to meet other people's expectations from emails and texts being answered within hours, if not minutes, to knowing that social media will report on our mistakes within seconds of an event occurring. It doesn't matter whether these stresses are within a business, within a Premier's office, or within our health system, there is still no excuse for unkind, disrespectful and bullying behaviour.

The Gathering of Kindness was unique and special. There are not too many opportunities where you have so many like-minded people gathered together in the one tent, talking about how to shift a culture from an old style hierarchical and somewhat intimidating system to a more respectful, engaging, open and honest system, which ensures patients are at its centre, while also providing for the needs of staff.

As a former health minister in the Tasmanian State Government, I met many good people dedicating their life's work to caring for others. But, I also met some staff broken by the behaviour of others within the system, I heard the excuses that change was not possible without dollars attached, I experienced passive resistance – "Just another health minister, we'll see her through." Or "What would she know, she's not a health professional!" I learnt change does not happen overnight, that you have to take people on a journey with you, but that change will happen with patience and persistence. After all, there is only so long the establishment can hold back the tide.

Change is happening. People are speaking out about behaviours they will no longer tolerate in their work place. People are being innovative and taking new ideas into the workplace to help shift thinking and behaviour. It was this sort of thinking that led Dr Catherine Crock to take the simple step of introducing music into the theatres and wards of the children's ward at the Royal Children's Hospital. The impact on the children, their parents and the staff was so positive that the Hush series was born. And what a delight it was to have both conference days interrupted by Professor Tony Gould playing pieces he composed for the 9th Hush CD. Watching Tony's fingers dance across the keys on the Steinway piano, within the gorgeous Duneira Estate House, surrounded by art works from Streeton to Warhol, provided for another example of the power of the arts in helping our minds to rest before going back into our discussions.

While there were many interesting stories told over the course of the two days of the conference, and none more so than the story of Assoc Prof Munjed Al Muderis, a man who risked his life on a boat to come to

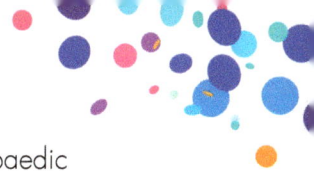

Australia as an asylum seeker, was detained in the Curtin Detention Centre, and is now an orthopaedic surgeon, the strongest message I got was from Prof. Billy O'Connor. What is it that allows some people to be more resilient than others? The importance of having a goal. The power of the embodiment of a goal can give you a cloak of self-confidence that enables you to cope with negativity, which otherwise could be hurtful and destructive. Of course, with a culture of kindness, this cloak is not so important for protection, but is an enabler for your talents to come to the fore to make a positive difference in someone else's life.

Thank you to Cath, Mary and team for bringing us together for such an enlightening and uplifting experience. #GoKindness

Building Kindness: The Next Steps

Robyn Klein and Peter Ellyard
Preferred Futures Institute

1. The Journey So Far

Dr Cath Crock has initiated and led a movement that has put the spotlight on hospital and health sector administrations and demanded that they confront and deal with a social cancer that has been growing within in their workplaces : workplace cruelty typified by bullying, intimidation, and other forms of threatening behaviour.   It is a paradox that hospitals and other health sector organisations - founded on and respected for practicing a culture of caring and healing - are being increasingly dominated by cruel work cultures that lead to increased bullying and intimidation, and from there onto increased patient and health worker illness . More of the same, business as usual, will only lead to further deterioration of this situation. New approaches are required.

2. Redefining the Mission

A conversation between Dr Crock and Pete resulted in Dr Crock redefining her mission. Instead of aspiring to deconstruct cruel behaviours such as bullying and intimidation in workplaces, she decided that it would be more productive to first imagine and second construct kind workplaces that practice and promote kind behaviours such as caring, nurturing and supporting.

The result of this strategic redefinition her aspirations led to a truly historic and amazing two day 'Gathering of Kindness' Conference on 31 March & 1 April 2016 , the story of which is being told by all of the contributors to this book .

3. Examining and Understanding Kindness

The 'Gathering of Kindness' was asked "What constitutes kindness?" We can't work to build any kindness movement without a shared understanding of what constitutes kindness and kind behaviour.

To us kindness has two elements in a simple equation:

* Kindness = the kind person (individual kindness) + the kind culture (collective kindness).

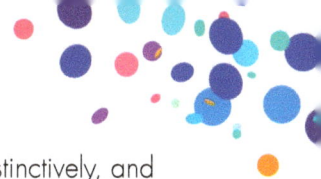

We should not seek to define the kind person more specifically. Everybody knows what this is instinctively, and if we try to do this we will divert ourselves into long and basically unproductive conversations around which disagreements can arise.

However, what we do need to say is that ending cruelty or bullying does not , of itself , result in the realisation of kindness and caring. Ending an undesirable entity does not mean it is automatically replaced by its desirable alternative. We must set out to consciously first imagine and second create this desirable alternative. Ending poverty does not create prosperity. Ending illness does not create wellness. Ending war does not create peace. Ending autocracy does not create democracy.

4. Kind and Cruel Behaviour

We also need to more thoroughly examine and understand kind and cruel behaviour.

- Kind behaviour can have many manifestations including caring, protecting and nurturing

- Cruel behaviour can have many manifestations including bullying, intimidation and threatening .

- A kind culture on the other hand could be described in many ways. We suggest to try to keep it as simple as possible.

- Therefore to us a kind culture = kind behaviour (individual kindness) + the golden rule (do unto others as you would have them do unto you) .

- We can have kind people in cruel cultures and cruel people in kind cultures. The strength and resilience of the dominant culture, kind or cruel, will determine whether the minority culture survives, grows and thrives, or dies.

5. Growing Kindness:

We consider that amongst the basic elements required for growing kindness are the following:

5a. Kindness and Trust .

Kindness is required for initiating trust in all relationships. And trust is, in turn, required to maintain kindness once it is established in a core culture. To trust another, each of us should ask and then answer yes to three core questions:

- Is the other honest?

- Is the other reliable?

- Is the other competent?

We cannot have a kind workplace or culture that does not embody trust.

5b. Kindness and Interdependence

Successful workplaces are interdependent workplaces. Interdependence can only grow if trust is first present. Interdependence can then be facilitated on a foundation of reciprocal respect and the shared seeking of win/win, not win/loss outcomes. Win/lose is perceived as cruel and win/win is perceived as kind. And respect and kindness are mutually reaffirming. Continuing win/loss will undermine and then destroy interdependent cultures and relationships and kindness will then be undermined by growing cruelty in workplaces.

5c. Kindness and Economic Productivity

Kind workplaces are economically productive workplaces. The Kindness Movement can contribute significantly to uplifting the economic productivity of hospital and indeed all workplaces.

Highly productive workplaces create synergistic outcomes (synergism is 2+2=5). The opposite to synergism is antagonism (antagonism is 2+2=3). Cruel workplaces are naturally antagonistic workplaces and therefore are unproductive workplaces as well.

6. Strategic Agenda

In the next stage of building the Kindness Movement we need to develop and implement detailed and practical strategies for:

- Transforming cruel cultures into kind cultures.

- Maintaining and strengthening kind cultures and increasing their resilience once kind cultures have developed

- Facilitating continuous innovation so that kindness continues to be uplifted through continuously creating emerging exemplary kind cultures.

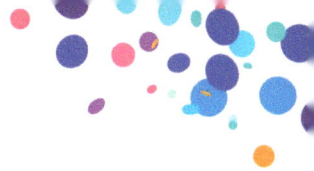

7. Our next personal steps - Pete Ellyard

Pete would like to take the kindness theme into other areas of concern.

Some of these are :

7a. Working to transform the current focus on Domestic Violence into one of Family Kindness, as a Kind Families Program. Focussing on the removal of domestic violence while not even dealing with lesser forms of cruelty such domestic bullying/intimidation is not likely to be successful. A Kind Family Vision, plus a strategy for realizing Family Kindness and for the promotion of Kind Family Ethics can, over time, undermine cruelty and violence in families. Helping victims and punishing those who practice domestic violence will not by itself, reduce domestic violence. A new Kind Families movement would create a positive alternative. And it is much more likely to succeed long -term.

7b. Transforming current anti-cyber bullying agendas into cyber-kindness agendas and seeking their implementation with interested partners.

7c. Focus on a redefining bullying in schools including redefining schoolyard cruelty, bullying and intimidation as a Kind Schools/School Kindness Program.

8. Our Next Personal steps - Robyn Klein

Robyn plans to deepen her work on uplifting both kindness and safety in relationships. She is interested in developing and implementing a toolkit for achieving this both in terms of kindness-to-self and kindness-to-other. She especially wishes to concentrate on increasing the adoption by more people of three key practices that can fortify kindness and safety in relationships namely:

- Mindfulness. This is a personal meditation practice, based on traditional Zen Buddhist Practice.

- Insight Dialogues. This is an interpersonal meditation practice. It brings the mindfulness and tranquillity of silent meditation directly into our experience with other people. As humans, we are relational beings; as we begin to wake up, clarity and freedom can illuminate our relationships with others (Gregory Kramer).

- Focusing. This shows how to pause the on-going situation and create a space for new possibilities for carrying forward. This practice shows how to apply open attention to something which is directly experienced but is not in words. Your body knows more about situations than you are explicitly aware of. This process enables you to get a bodily feel for the 'more' that is happening in any situation. From that bodily feel comes small steps that can lead toward resolution (Gene Gendelin).

Caring for ourselves so we can care for others

Katrina Hall
Eastern Health

It seems we have a Kindness deficit. Bullying and poor behaviour occur in healthcare organizations on a daily basis. This is really important because not only does it lead to misery, humiliation and suffering for staff, it can also lead to errors in patient management. The Gathering of Kindness saw an awesome collection of people get together to brainstorm and plan ways to address the Kindness deficit. We began by watching the play "Hear me" by Alan Hopgood AM. This excruciating play struck me with the pain of the mother and the young doctor, suffered as a result of poor staff behaviour. Doctors are too often blamed, but we are all part of this problem and we can all be part of the solution.

Using a familiar improvement methodology I asked myself what the causes of unkind behaviour might be.

1. Physical stressors - tiredness, hunger, pain

2. Emotional stressors - stress, anxiety, sadness, frustration

3. Professional culture – valuing outcome over process, responsibility for patient outcomes

4. No fail-safe system – doctors not allowed to make mistakes, no double-check, fear of litigation

5. Voice of consumer not heard – patient not given or allowed responsibility for decisions, not valued as team member, dismissed or discounted

Further exploration suggests the following root causes:

1. Poor rostering and culture, excessive overtime, no protected meal time or time off

2. Historic behaviour, toughness rather than self-care or team work, frequent rotations

3. Poor behaviour accepted, short term contracts, visiting staff

4. Historically punitive culture

5. Historically patient and family voice not relevant,

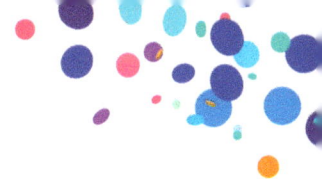

Actions to address these root cause:

1. Develop General Staff Health standards including healthy rosters, healthy eating and protected time off

2. Promote emotional self-care through optional reflection leave (an hour or a day); provide dedicated staff reflection places (as we do for patients)

3. Embed all staff in teams and teach teamwork and positive communication

4. Establish regular interprofessional team meetings, case conferences; challenge the historic culture

5. Shift primary responsibility for care and treatment decisions to patients and carers; document 'primary decision maker' in every patient file.

This roadmap is based on the thoughts of just one person. It needs to be workshopped by a diverse group to strengthen and develop the ideas; but it is a starting point.

We are all capable of unkindness and this is more likely to happen when we are tired, stressed or in pain. Whether you're a relative in ED with a loved one, an inpatient in a mental health unit or a doctor on a 12 hour shift, human factors affect behaviour. If we truly want to improve behaviour in hospitals I think we should begin by creating a truly caring culture. As leaders demonstrate their care for staff through healthy staff policies, staff will be better able to provide the best care for patients.

Well cared for staff will always provide the best patient care.

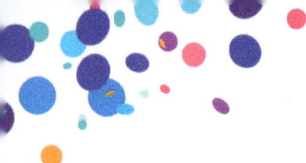

A/Prof Munjed Al Muderis
Orthopaedic surgeon

"We are all born of different colours and places.

We didn't choose our race, ethnicity, background or the faith to which we were born.

We must remember to treat each other the way we wish to be treated: with respect, tolerance and kindness".

The unspoken hierarchy

Luigi Zolio

MBBS/BMedSc(Hons) student, Monash University
President, Monash University Medical Undergraduates' Society

In order to be kind, we must flip the unspoken hierarchy.

Conferences can be a daunting environment for people who are only at the beginning of their careers. We don't always feel comfortable speaking up in front of our seniors, and at the beginning of the Gathering this was how I felt. In a small discussion group, I was eager to hear the perspectives and wisdom of those more senior to me, but I chose to refrain from sharing, unsure of what I was able to contribute. It so then happened that a senior person in the group took an admirable step in leadership. He acknowledged that our group discussion dynamics reinforced an unspoken seniority hierarchy – only the most senior members were talking, and the juniors passively listening. He called on himself and others to listen out to the quieter members of our group, and kindly encouraged the latter to feel comfortable speaking up, for we definitely had important contributions to make.

I chose to accept this opportunity, hoping that what I could add might be valuable. My contribution was to share my experiences of attending multidisciplinary meetings in hospitals as a medical student. Despite those meetings being a forum for nursing and allied health staff to share their insights with each other and with doctors, I rarely saw anybody other than a doctor speaking. I always wondered what the other staff got out of those meetings if their knowledge and insights were not acknowledged. Further, to sit on chair at the table was an unspoken exercise in authority and power, a privilege to which only a select few were entitled. As medical students, if we had arrived early and found a chair, we would give it up at the first opportunity for someone else. I recounted that in my eyes, this was an unfortunate acknowledgement of the already accepted hierarchy within our hospitals which disempowered many professionals on a daily basis. It only served to drown out the voices of the least empowered, and seemed to counter-act the purpose of a multi-disciplinary meeting. No wonder only doctors felt comfortable speaking.

One week on from the Gathering, I had the sobering opportunity to witness the concept of the implicit hierarchy be exemplified within the medical students' society, of which I am the president. I stepped into my role with the aim to treat my fellow committee members as my equals, and to be approachable and kind in my demeanour. This was something which I also asked my fellow senior members to practise in their roles. Nonetheless, our full

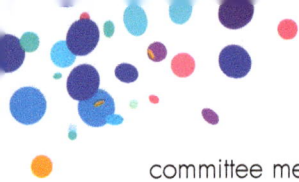

committee meetings are an incredibly daunting environment, with over fifty members attending and all of whom vary in their roles and seniority within the course. I can recall my days as a second year student in a junior committee role where putting my hand up to speak made my heart race.

And so, just before the start of our meeting, two of our junior committee members asked our secretary whether it would be ok for them to sit near the front. "Of course you may, you are welcome to sit anywhere" replied the secretary, caught off guard by the concept that somebody thought they needed to ask him where they could sit. Were we such a hierarchical group that people felt like they could not sit in certain places, just like at the hospital?

We later reflected that as senior committee members, it was our job to actively flip the hierarchy upside down, just as my senior group member had done at the Gathering. While in our minds we may with good intent perceive others as our equals, this is not necessarily reciprocated by the least empowered, who naturally perceive themselves as inferior. Even when our actions aim to project kindness onto others through our demeanour, actions such as inviting our junior members to sit near us, or prompts for them to share their views can be far more powerful. To be kind can mean to empower someone, to give them confidence and a sense of importance. To be kind may mean to remove ourselves from our pedestals and engage others with humility.

Anthem for Hush

Tony Gould

Acts of kindness are never in vain, even if we don't see their impact

Michael Greco

CEO, Patient Opinion Australia

We often hear that it is love that makes the world go round. I have to agree with that. Those smitten with love, and many of our songs are about this, will know the experience of 'being in love'. However, love is more than just a feeling or 'being smitten'. Love is a choice and it is acts of kindness that operationalise our love.

That choice is refined in times of hardship. Many of us, if not all of us, go through some tough times. Whatever the reason for these difficulties, that is when we have to dig deep and continue to make the choice of offering kindness to those around us. As mentioned at the Gathering of Kindness conference, it was Victor Frankl who wrote the book called *Man's search for meaning*. He was in a Nazi concentration camp and noticed that those who survived were usually those who had a goal in life, a purpose, in particular a meaning for living. They made the choice, despite the atrocious conditions, to stand firm and stay strong to their values.

I'd like to share a brighter story about my work as a Franciscan friar some years ago now. I was involved with a youth outreach centre based in Paddington, Sydney. One of my roles was to just offer kindness and friendship to the troubled youth in that area, and in surrounding areas such as Kings Cross. I was asked one day to talk to an older teenager who had been badly beaten while working as a sex-worker at the Cross. He was quite an intelligent young man and it was felt that it would be good if he could somehow engage with the educational system again, such as attending a TAFE course. So we spent a couple hours a week just chatting about things, doing walks from Bronte beach to Bondi, and even occasionally going for a surf.

After some months, I was posted to Melbourne where I completed my theological studies and assisted the Pentridge prison chaplain. I wasn't sure what eventuated with the young man that I 'walked with' in Sydney. However, some years later I was working for the Royal Australian College of General Practitioners and met a woman who was a social worker as part of a project on preventing youth suicide. She too worked in Sydney at the time I was there. Being a small world, she also knew the teenager that I had 'walked with'.

What took me by total surprise was that she told me that he was now married and doing really fine. Wow, I was 'bowled over' knowing that this young man had turned things around.

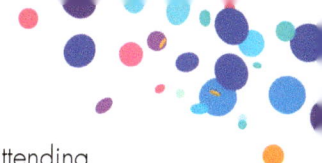

Now, it should be said that I was only one small part of this young man's journey. He was also attending various services such as counselling and other social services. However, I don't think we can ever underestimate the importance of showing kindness to others.

And the way we show kindness is unique to all of us. We have been gifted in different ways. What we have to discover is how we best do that. But I can assure you that no act of kindness is ever wasted. And sometimes, if we are lucky, we hear about the impact of what we have tried to do. Just like the young man in this story.

Gwenda – God's gift to our family.

Max Dumais

www.aheadofthegame.com.au

As my kids were growing through adolescence, we often had a visitor from an old person's home around the corner. It was of particular interest because it was the original Salvation Army facility where the first moving picture in Australia was shot.

Gwenda's habit was to walk up and down our street knocking on doors and asking for a few dollars for cigarettes. I have no idea how well she got on in other places, but it was my habit to invite her in, and aside from the money she asked for, offer her a stash of groceries that we kept especially for her.

My children were not impressed by this largesse. They found Gwenda's body odour offensive and they considered her to be bludging on the kindness of others like a hobo. They were dismayed at the efforts that were taken to ensure there would always be a pack of her favourite biscuits and the bottle of her preferred cordial kept on hand for her arrival.

To me this was a deliberate lesson in life, and my comeback to them was couched in the words of Christ, "When you do this to the least of my brethren then you do it to me" – but they found that a bit of a stretch. This was a lesson deeply ingrained to me through my time walking in the footsteps of St Francis as a monk in his Order. Though I did find it a lop-sided compliment to my worldly adjustment that my kids found that part of my life so hard to imagine!

Imagine my own pleasant surprise to hear each of my children, as adults and in their own lives, at various times recount the salutary experiences that Gwenda had bought to our family to others within my hearing.

We were all a little sad when the news filtered through that Gwenda had passed on and would no longer be knocking on our door. I am grateful to her and I think my children today appreciate the opportunity she presented in learning the joy of giving and the significance of this message we, ourselves, were receiving through her.

It's not necessary to be moved by Christian, or even religious, reasons to reach out to others – even those by whom we might be offended or even disgusted. There is, however, a joy in the kindness of giving we can discover and it is its own reward no matter how large or small our efforts, provided there is a real human connection and intent.

Being GOOD vs. Being NICE

Dr. Avnesh Ratnanesan (Avi)

CEO, Energesse
Customer-Centred Healthcare

"Living up to an image that you have of yourself or that other people have of you is inauthentic living." ~ Eckhart Tolle, A New Earth: Awakening to Your Life's Purpose

As I was sitting at a café on Saturday morning, psyching myself up for another day of writing a chapter in my book on transforming the healthcare experience, I glanced at the daily paper. I do not spend too much time with newspapers these days, as it is often filled with irrelevant negativity and I prefer to get my news elsewhere. However, whilst sipping a cup of my favourite tea - English Breakfast - I came across an article interviewing a famous model.

Miranda Kerr was quoted as saying "There's a difference between being nice and good, I consider myself a good person. And I think people perceive me to be nice as in, 'Oh, she's nice,' but being a good person, knowing your strengths and working towards those strengths, and encouraging those around you to do the same, that's a good person. A nice person will sit back and go, 'Oh yes, OK, no worries, yes.' A nice person is a yes person, whereas a good person is a person who accepts their responsibility in things and moves forward. He or she constantly evolves and isn't afraid to say no, challenge someone or be honest."

Most people would not expect such profound words from a model, but indeed her thoughts are backed by scientific research. The Psychology Foundation of Canada reports that one important aspect of your personal self-esteem is feeling that you have a 'voice' — that you have the right to be listened to and heard in a way that helps you have some control over what happens in your life. When you speak up and stand up for yourself, you are, in effect, saying to yourself and the world, "I am a significant person whose ideas and words are worthy of respect."

So you can be nice, but also be good as well. Being good and kind to your authentic self allows you to be successful in your endeavours to champion change and improvements our healthcare system whilst growing, rather than diminishing, your self worth.

Reflections on empathy

Don Campbell
Professor of Medicine, Monash University
Program Director, General Medicine, Monash Health

We live in our own heads. We think and express our thoughts as a series of endless conversations in our own minds. How do we construct our realities? Our self-talk shapes our view of the universe.

A kindly worldview is constructed in our thoughts on the basis of seeing those with whom we interact as kin, hence kinship and kindness. Are people kind to each other? Can we learn kindness? Kindness has to be a disposition, a way of being.

What has this got to do with healthcare or medicine?

Healthcare at its heart is a set of privileged relations between two people mediated by a conversation. Trust, essential to the relationship, is constructed through conversation, and carries with it an implicit obligation that the healthcare provider will act in the best interests of the person seeking their assistance.

To be kind we have to see our relations with others as kin. We can't do this if we see people, particularly those with whom we have a professional relationship within health care, as a generalized other.

Empathy is an English translation of a German word Einfuhlung literally 'feeling into' or the ability to recognize and share the emotions of another. Empathy involves seeing someone else's situation from their own perspective, and sharing their emotions, including distress.

Empathy is the foundation of the obligations upon the healthcare provider. Empathy is implicit in the relationship between the healthcare professional and the person whom they serve. This relationship is one where the balance of responsibility for decision making is contextual.

Doctors in particular, will need to re-learn and ensure that future generations of doctors see empathy enacted, both cognitive and affective. Ultimately Doctors are social beings whose identity as a health care professional lives in the conversation and the acts which follow, on the basis of trust. This is the privilege afforded to doctors. Ideally they will model empathy in conversation with those people who seek their assistance, whom they serve.

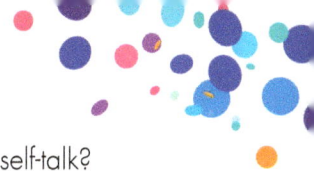

The self-talk we have is the only means we have to change our culture. How can we change our self-talk? Arguably, the easiest way is to practice it in our interactions or conversations. We will only change our (healthcare) culture by changing our self talk, and to do this we will have to change the way that we healthcare professionals talk, with each other and with those who seek our assistance as patients.

The crisis in medical education at present reflects the transition from its former basis as an altruistic calling with implicit contextual relational responsibilities, mediated through trust established in conversation based on empathy and kinship, to a set of contractual technical transactions which are no longer grounded in context or community, hence these narrow transactional responsibilities are no longer mediated through kindness, kinship or connectedness.

The restoration of kindness as a state of being central to healthcare will require assumptions to be made explicit and requisite behaviours will need to be modeled and taught in context as a set of empathic relationships and responsibilities.

Stories and enactments are essential to the way that people learn the importance of kindness as the basis for a model of healthcare as a set of actions built on trust mediated through conversation. This is why a gathering of kindness is so important as a first step to creating a community to support the restoration of kindness to its rightful place as the foundation of our healthcare system.

An image of kindness

Marlene Gojanovic

This photo was taken in Hawaii on the North Shore. I like this picture because similar to the workplace, I think it demonstrates quite well the importance of sharing kindness and respect in the surf. Surfing is a much more enjoyable and fun experience with people who share the waves in a kind and respectful way.

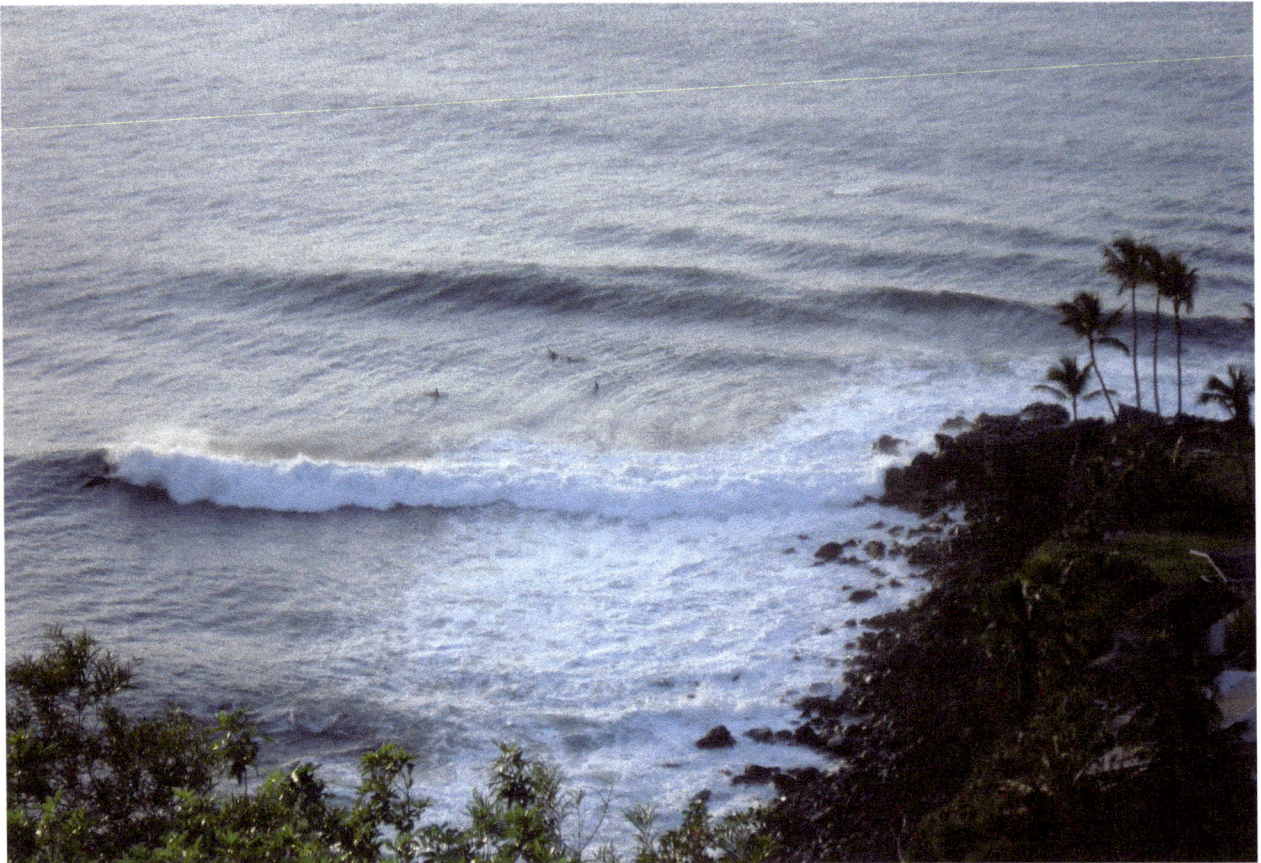

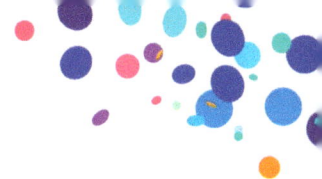

The true measure

Jenny Lee Seedsman

The true measure of a person is how they handle personal interactions in a stressed environment. Anybody can be kind when life is going well, but the real person is revealed in how they behave when life gets tough. This is especially true in how people deal with those more vulnerable around them, the sick, the very young, the elderly, the disabled and especially the animals around us - those with little, or no voice. At some point each and every one of us has to stop, reflect and ask ourselves "How much of our own pain and angst are we passing on to the next person?" When is it time to stop the continuum?

Be kind to one's selfie

Simon Pase

Hurt people hurt people. So, if we're the people that fix hurt people, why haven't we fixed this problem yet? I heard so many reasons at the Gathering of Kindness. Opinions from learned people. Everyday people. They even asked me to speak, which speaks volumes about the courage of the organisers. Heads nodded. Some painful wounds were reopened. When it sounded so true, we laughed. When it sounded like it shouldn't be true, we cried.

Truth be told we've had these conversations already, haven't we? I know we have. I've overheard them, contributed to them, and when they're particularly hard, I've even evaded them.

The conversation I'm trying to have more often about Kindness is with me. I hit the replay button and wonder what my words, actions and inactions mean for those around me. Did I listen? Did I keep an open mind? Was I reasonable or unreasonable? Did I say I'm sorry? Did I forgive?

Am I having this conversation every day? Of course not! Most days I'm flat out asking myself why I've paid $3.50 for coffee (trust me, in Italy coffee is a third the price and at least three times better).

It is a conversation I need to have every now and then though. So do you I reckon. You'll help make others kinder for it. So I've come up with a concept for an app that you can use as regularly as you drink a coffee, and hopefully as awakening. It's a mirror we can hold up to ourselves just once a day, once a week, or even once a month.

THE KINDNESS MIRROR   BY SIMON PASE

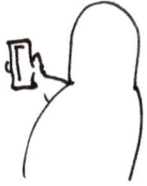

A SMARTPHONE APP

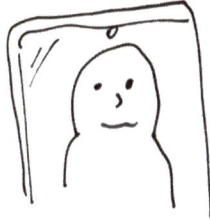

FRONT CAMERA ACTS AS A MIRROR

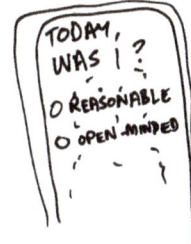

TODAY, WAS I?
- REASONABLE
- OPEN-MINDED

PERTINENT QUESTIONS FORM A SELF-REFLECTION (OVER AN IMAGE OF ONE'S SELF!)

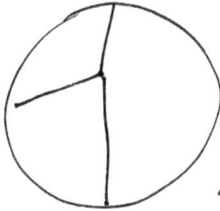

RESULTS ...

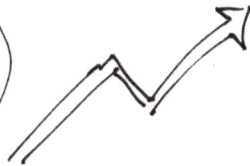

ANONYMISED
+
AGGREGATED
+
SHARED ACROSS THE HEALTH SECTOR ...

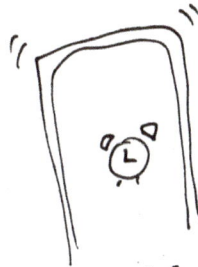

REMINDS YOU IF YOU HAVEN'T "LOOKED IN THE MIRROR LATELY"

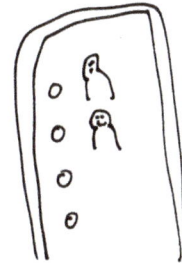

TAP A CONTACT TO THANK THEM FOR BEING A TRULY KIND HUMAN BEING!

Kindness Change

Jitka Jilich

Pre...
Real change is...
Organisational change?
Macro ... systemic?
Must come from the top to make a real difference?
It's 'all' about management ... if they're not on board ...
Forget it ... Nothing will be different!

At...
 A GATHERING OF KINDNESS
100 people together ... thinking and sharing ... kindness
What it looks like ... What it 'could' look like

Harnessing kindness
such a simple concept
... isn't it?
... isn't it??
The first spark ... one individual ... could be 'me' ... 'you' .... 'together'???
Sparks ignite
Agency ... influence
Acts of kindness ... being kind
Simple?
A smile, gesture, touch, a conversation, a statement
Congratulations!
How can I help you?
You're amazing!
Caring ... caring spaces

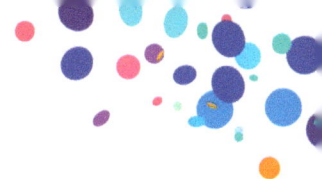

The KTag ... Kindness tag ...
Passing kindness on.
It really is simple.

Infectious
The water wheel ... gathering momentum
I'm feeling inspired ... uplifted

Back at work
... suddenly luminous ... why didn't I see it before
People ...
Generosity
Respect
Care
It's already here
Let's gather, sew, grow!!
Kindness change

Start now

Kate Bowles

It's 9pm when we're flung into the hospital. There's a bed, and blue curtains, and a monitor. I'm holding all the things, trying to remember who to call, where the keys are, whether anything was left in the ambulance by mistake.

And that's when I notice I'm still wearing my Gathering of Kindness t-shirt, with its big blue button: Be Kind.

Refugee and advocate Munjed Al Muderis explains that sometimes people who learn English later in adult life become abrupt speakers who speak in commands rather than requests. In this moment of rushing silence I notice that this is what the t-shirt does for us all. It's an instruction to be kind, an order, a slogan.

But the world we are trying to imagine differently is one in which good process isn't a response to order. It's a world that offers the right physical space and enough human time for each of us to react compassionately because that is who we are, not because that is what we were told we must do.

I am committed to this as a teacher, as a patient, and as a patient advocate. I believe that it is in the gift of patients to act compassionately even in difficult moments, and to extend kindness to those who are trying to help when they are themselves desperately tired, unsure what to do, and have so many reasons to be frustrated with their work.

And so now here I am, sitting with my demanding t-shirt in an emergency department, supporting a late-night admission that has been chaotic, confusing, and frightening. And as I'm watching the monitor's erratic parallels wandering across the screen, I'm thinking: who will see me and wonder in this moment what this t-shirt means to me? What can kindness mean here, in this place?

There's a man in a bed whose late-night emergency is an end of life crisis. His son is with him. He is familiar with his cancer and he's calmly advising doctors and nurses one by one about the state of things. There's no bed, no one is sure what to do next. Nurses are drawn to him, they hang out with him to hold his hand. He jokes about his situation, and his son rolls his eyes.

He's alert and clear and in pain, and I watch him taking care of everyone who comes his way. In his hands, the hospital place becomes a hospitable space. He has achieved the miracle of kindness that all of us want to be part of.

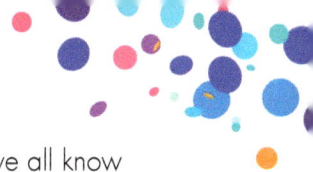

To create kindness in healthcare we need first to understand how well humans can do this, how we all know how to mind each other well, in even the extreme situations.

It's 3am. I'm sitting in a plastic chair, leaning on a bed and resting my cheek on a hospital pillow, listening to the monitor's sympathetic investigation of a heart that's still somehow beating, wearing a t-shirt. I am saying to myself: remember, you are here too.

Start now.

celebrate kind acts, not kind people.

As the editor of this Anthology, I had the privilege of getting to know the wonderful variety of perspectives that came out of the Gathering of Kindness in intimate detail. You don't just read every submission once. You read them multiple times, closely, word by word. And through that process, my definition of what kindness is, my understanding of the different experiences that people have had, and my assumptions of what was 'to be learnt' from the Gathering were challenged time and time again.

This book makes it clear there are infinite ways to be kind. There will never be a single definition of kindness, it's not something that can be adequately codified or accurately defined. It varies situationally, culturally, and individually. We will continue to learn, all through our lives, what kindness is and how to offer kindness to others. We will get it wrong, sometimes! And this can be disheartening, particularly when we think our intentions are good. But persevere, learn from the experience, and try again. So many more times you will get it right.

Kindness begets kindness, so celebrate kind acts whenever you see them. And don't withhold praise for a kind act from an unkind person, because in that moment they proved that kindness truly does exist within them. Humans like to label. It is an unfortunate habit of ours! And in this case, it's all too easy to settle on the notion that some people are kind, while others are not. But in doing so, we take away the opportunity for everyone to show kindness. Celebrate kind acts, not kind people.

The moment where the idea for the Gathering of Kindness shifted from "Let's solve the problem of bullying" to "Let's create a culture of kindness" was a life-changing one for everyone involved. Dr Dan Diamond, Director of the medical response for hurricane Katrina, talks about the Law of Target Fixation in his book 'Beyond Resilience':

"Where we look is also contagious to other people. Think about the last time you pass somebody on the street and they were looking up in the air. You couldn't help but glance to see where they were looking. The same thing happens in the workplace. It is all too easy to get sucked into negativity. On the contrary, if you keep your gaze locked in the direction that you want to go, in the direction you want to move your team, you are much more likely to succeed."

The healthcare industry has spent as long time focused on bullying, and seemingly made very little progress moving away from it. Perhaps that's an example of Dan's observation in action; you go where you look. So we resolve to look towards kindness. To look in the direction of love and compassion and forgiveness and all those intangible qualities that make being human so important.

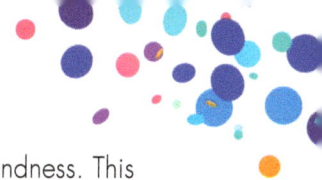

Thank you for reading this Anthology, and for your kind acts. For this is not a movement 'about' kindness. This is a movement 'of' kindness. There are no entrance exams, or certificates of authenticity. The price of entry is simply one kind act, and then another, and another.

Mish Phillips
Editor

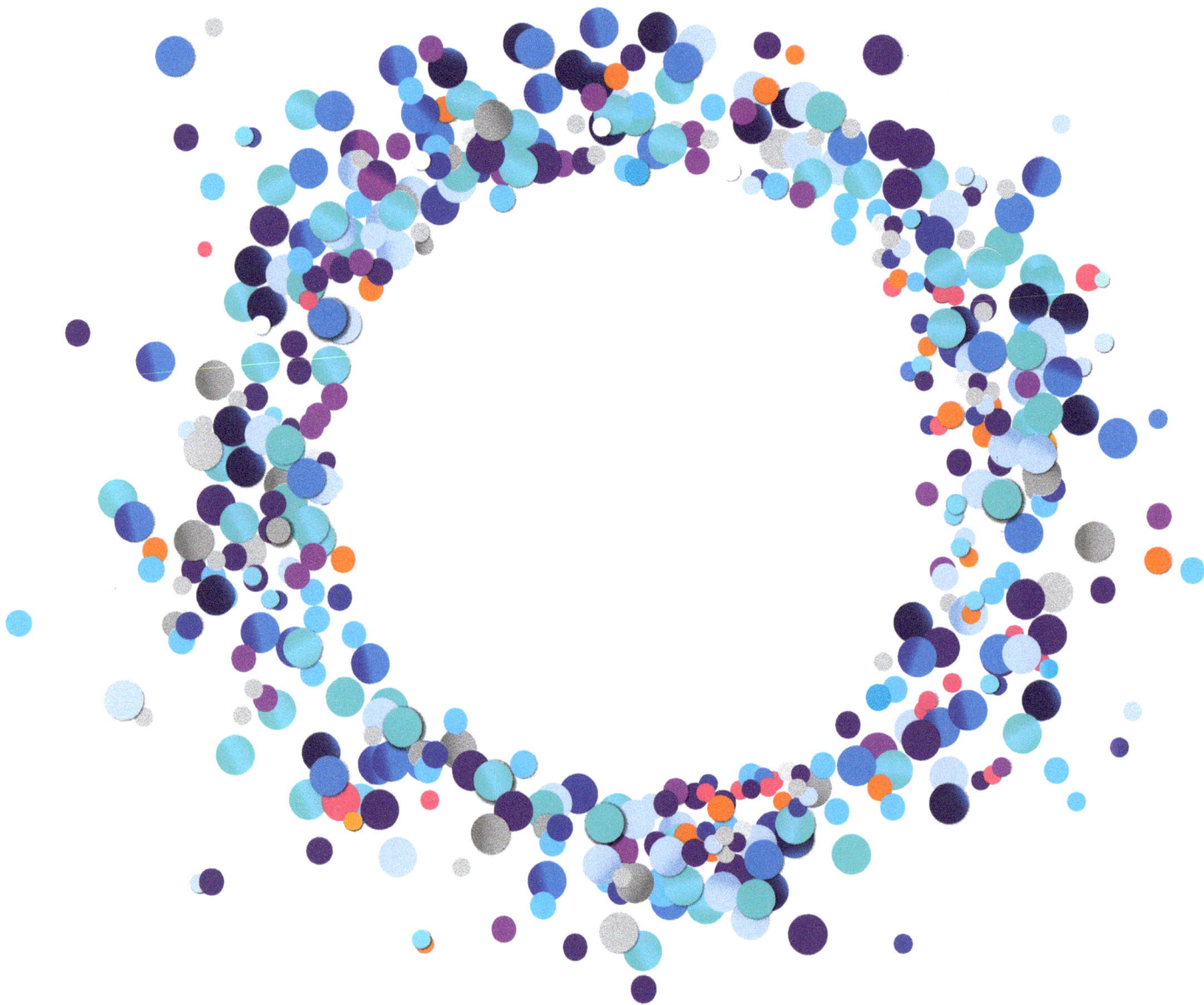

www.ingramcontent.com/pod-product-compliance
Lightning Source LLC
Chambersburg PA
CBHW051612030426
42334CB00035B/3500